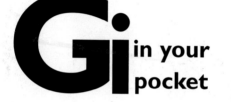

G in your pocket

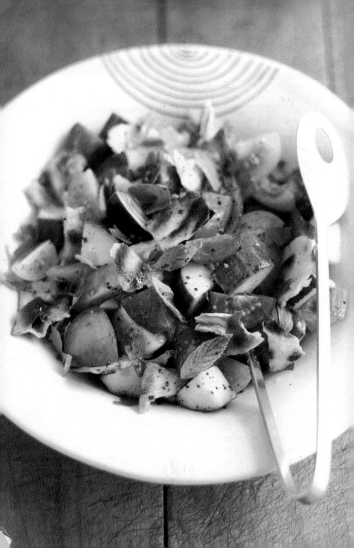

Gi in your pocket

Dr Barbara Wilson

NEW
HOLLAND

First published in 2006 by New Holland Publishers (UK) Ltd
London • Cape Town • Sydney • Auckland

Garfield House
86-88 Edgware Road
London W2 2EA
www.newhollandpublishers.com

80 McKenzie Street
Cape Town 8001
South Africa

Level 1, Unit 4
14 Aquatic Drive
Frenchs Forest, NSW 2086
Australia

218 Lake Road
Northcote
Auckland
New Zealand

1 3 5 7 9 10 8 6 4 2

ISBN 13: 978 1 84537 488 4
ISBN 10: 1 84537 488 6

Senior Editor: Corinne Masciocchi
Design: Sue Rose
Photography: Stuart West, Shona Wood, John Freeman and Ryno
Editorial Direction: Rosemary Wilkinson
Production: Hazel Kirkman

Reproduction by Pica Digital PTE Ltd, Singapore
Printed and bound by Star Standard Industries, Singapore

contents

introduction *6*

introduction

Don't you find that every time you open a magazine or newspaper, the latest and greatest dieting secret is being revealed? Get the body you're after in three weeks, perfect your workout in 10 minutes or drop a dress size overnight! Diets and weight-loss plans seem to come and go and the next big thing is always just around the corner.

But did you know that the GI (glycaemic index) revolution has been slowly gaining momentum for 25 years? In 1981, Dr David Jenkins and colleagues at the University of Toronto carried out a study to determine the effect that different foods have on the blood glucose levels of healthy volunteers in relation to glucose[1]. They found that different foods caused the volunteers' blood glucose levels to rise at varying rates, and so the glycaemic index was born!

The new system ranked carbohydrate foods into low, medium and high categories, depending on the impact they had on blood glucose levels. Low-GI foods were categorized as those with a value of 55 or less, medium-GI was categorized as 56–69 and high-GI foods were those with values of 70 or over, while the reference standard, glucose, had a value of 100. It was initially hoped that this new system would help in the management of diabetes mellitus, a condition in which the body cannot effectively, if at all, regulate blood glucose levels. But it is now thought that the implications of the glycaemic index are more wide-ranging than diabetes management alone. The use of the glycaemic index has been proposed to be effective in the management of weight problems, heart disease, behavioural disorders and even in enhancing athletic performance[2-4].

It has also been found that swapping foods high on the glycaemic index for those with lower values can help prevent the development of type 2 diabetes. This condition can develop when the body becomes less sensitive to insulin, the hormone produced in response to an increase in blood sugars. When high-GI foods are eaten, a greater insulin response is triggered; lower GI foods cause a less dramatic release of insulin, which the body is better able to cope with in the long term. Choosing low- over high-GI foods can also help limit hypoglycaemic episodes in those with type 1 diabetes[5] (see page 31 for more information).

Heart disease risk is another area where following a low GI diet can be beneficial. Leeds writes[6] that individuals following a low GI diet have lower total cholesterol and lower LDL cholesterol (low density lipoprotein cholesterol – the unhealthy type of cholesterol), and reduced levels of certain markers of disease, when compared to those following a high GI diet.

But the most universally popular reason for following the principles of the glycaemic index is weight control. We've been told in recent years that fat is the enemy and carbohydrates are our friends. Then we heard that carbs were out and fat was back on the menu! And now we're being told that carbs are good again – but only the right kind of carbs. What are we to believe!

Well, there are many ways in which eating primarily low-GI foods is beneficial for weight loss. These types of food promote satiety, or the feeling of fullness, they help the body control the amount of insulin produced and they help ensure that insulin continues to function efficiently and effectively.

High GI diets, on the other hand, can enhance weight gain, even when low- and high GI diets of the same calorie level are compared. High GI diets promote weight gain around the abdomen (visceral adiposity) and increase fat production through a higher concentration of the enzymes that promote fat storage. Waist size also increases as the GI of the diet rises[7].

So, these sound like fairly convincing reasons to make sure that most of the foods you eat have a low ranking on the glycaemic index.

If you have diabetes, eating low-GI foods can help you make good carb choices, stabilizing your blood sugars and insulin levels and help prevent hypos. If a close relative already has diabetes, following a low GI diet can help reduce your risk of developing the condition.

If you have heart disease or problems with high cholesterol, the principles of GI can help. And if you want to lose weight, maintain weight loss or finally get off that dieting roller-coaster, GI could be the answer you're looking for!

The great thing about low GI eating is that it's easy. You don't have to say goodbye to an entire food group, eat grapefruit with every meal or only eat certain foods at certain times. Following the principles of GI means making simple, everyday choices. Cut down on the amount of high-GI foods that you eat and replace these with lower GI alternatives. It's as easy as swapping sticky rice for basmati rice, creamed potatoes for boiled new potatoes in their skins or changing your morning breakfast cereal from corn flakes to porridge or 100% bran.

Once you're aware of which foods have higher and lower GI values, you can make better nutritional choices in one easy step! And your life doesn't have to revolve around low-GI foods. You can still eat high-GI foods occasionally, since when these are combined with low-GI options, the overall GI value of the meal is reduced. These easy, day-to-day decisions could be the single greatest thing you can do to improve your diet and your health.

Dr Debora wilson

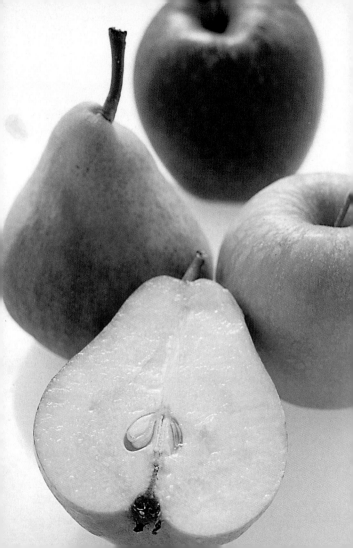

how does it work?

How do I recognize low-GI foods?

So, we've seen that the glycaemic index is a system of ranking carbohydrates but what does that actually mean? And what exactly are carbohydrates?

Carbohydrates are one of three macronutrients found in food, the other two being protein and fat. All of these macronutrients provide energy and this is expressed in terms of kilocalories (more often abbreviated to 'calories') and kilojoules (kJ).

Carbohydrates and protein each provide 4 calories (16.8 kJ) per gram while fat provides 9 calories (37.8 kJ) per gram. Alcohol is another source of energy often found in our diets and each gram of alcohol provides us with 7 calories (29.4 kJ).

Simple and complex carbohydrates

There are two main categories of carbohydrates: **simple** and **complex** carbs. Simple carbohydrates have basic chemical structures that can be relatively easily digested and broken down, while complex carbohydrates have more complicated structures that tend to take longer to digest. These categories can be further split into more descriptive groups based on chemical structure.

All carbohydrates are made up from building blocks known as saccharides. The simplest carbs – sugars – have only one saccharide. These are known as **monosaccharides** and are glucose, fructose and galactose.

Sugars made up from two monosaccharides are still classed as simple sugars and these are called **disaccharides**. These are maltose (glucose + glucose), sucrose (glucose + fructose) and lactose (glucose + galactose).

Complex carbohydrates are made up from many (more than 10) saccharides formed into more complicated structures, some straight chains and others branching, and are known as **polysaccharides**. They are found in:

STARCH

♥ starchy foods are those we think of as 'fillers' – bread, potatoes, rice and pasta, as well as beans and vegetables, especially root vegetables

♥ for better nutrition, we should try to choose wholegrain or unrefined starchy foods whenever possible as these have higher fibre content than refined versions.

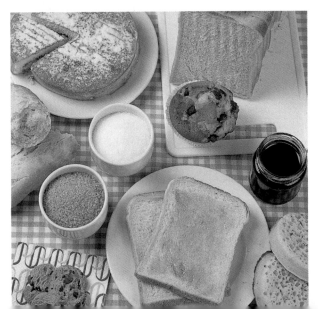

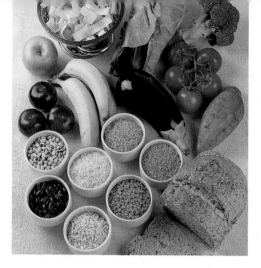

DIETARY FIBRE, OR 'ROUGHAGE'

♥ fibre is so complex in structure that it cannot be digested at all and so it doesn't provide energy (other simple and complex carbs provide 4 calories per gram)

♥ the presence of fibre slows digestion of the foods it is contained in

♥ insoluble fibre is the type found in wheat bran, wholegrains, the skins of fruit and vegetables and seeds. Its job is to absorb water, bulking up the contents of the digestive system and protecting the health of the digestive system. It also provides food for gut bacteria.

♥ soluble fibre is found in oats, legumes, brown rice, fruit and vegetables and potatoes. It dissolves to form a gel that can trap cholesterol, lowering unhealthy LDL cholesterol.

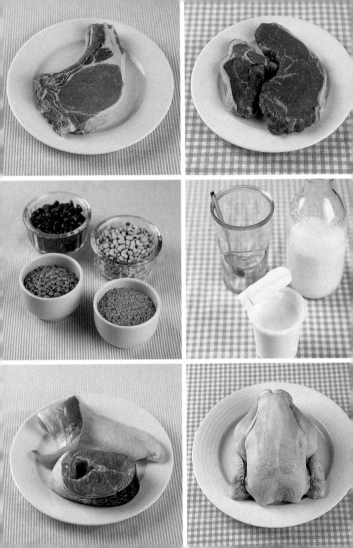

SUGAR ALCOHOLS OR POLYOLS
♥ used as artificial sweeteners

♥ they provide fewer than the usual 4 calories per gram of digestible carbohydrates as they are not fully broken down in the body.

Carbohydrates are our body's preferred source of energy as these are easily broken down into glucose, a simple sugar that circulates around our body in the blood stream. Protein and fat, on the other hand, have functions in the body other than energy production and so are only used as energy sources when carbohydrate isn't an option.

So, when we eat foods containing carbohydrates, they are broken down into basic glucose molecules. These are taken up by the bloodstream to circulate around the body and provide energy where it's needed.

Now, it would seem to make sense if the monosaccharides were broken down most quickly and had highest GI values through to the polysaccharides being broken down slowly and having low GI values. But this isn't always the case.

As we can see in the table on page 17, GI values within each of the categories of saccharides vary between low, medium and high. This makes it difficult to make a best guess about the GI value of a food based on its structure alone.

One thing we can be sure of, though, is that the presence of fibre or sugar alcohols will lower the GI of a food. Fibre slows the overall digestion of food and can check the rate at which glucose

◀ *Proteins are broken down into amino acids and are used for growth and repair. Protein can also be used as an energy source when no carbohydrate is available.*

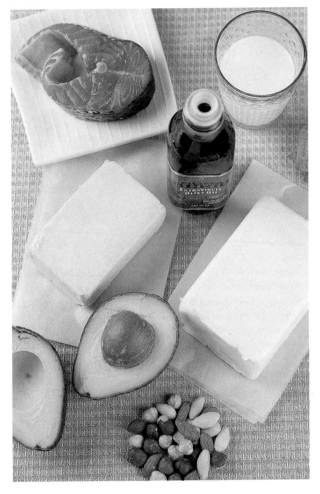

Category of sugar	Type of sugar	GI (approx values)
monosaccharides	glucose fructose galactose	high (100) low (19) lower (*)
disaccharides	maltose sucrose lactose	high (105) medium (68) low (46)
polysaccharides	amylopectin amylose dietary fibre	higher (*) lower (*) very low / none
sugar alcohols	polyols	very low / none

(*) *There are no GI values available for galactose, amylopectin or amylose.*

makes it from food into the bloodstream. The body has to work harder and for longer to release energy from food that is rich in fibre than food that is low in fibre.

Artificial sweeteners made with sugar alcohols also have lower GI values. This is because they are not recognized by the body as carbohydrates and are not metabolized as such.

Food manufacturers hoping to tap into the low-GI market can now re-formulate their foods to lower their GI value by replacing some of the sugars with the polysaccharide polydextrose (a type of fibre that isn't available to the body) or sugar alcohols, such as lactitol or xylitol.

◀ *While fat has a bad reputation, it does have a lot of uses in the body: it is a carrier for the fat-soluble vitamins A, D, E and K, it's used in the structure of cell walls, it's needed for hormone production, and essential fatty acids are vital for nerve and brain development. Of course, fat is also a source of energy.*

Why does fructose have a low GI value?

Simple sugars that are broken down quickly and absorbed as glucose often have higher GI values. For example, glucose itself is often used as a reference with a value of 100. Maltose has an even higher GI of 105 while sucrose and lactose have lower values of around 60 and 45, respectively.

However, the monosaccharide fructose has a GI value of only 11–24. As a monosaccharide, you might expect this to be much higher, so why is it so low?

The answer is that fructose, and other sugars to differing degrees, are not broken down in the digestive tract and absorbed directly

---

WHAT ROLE DOES INSULIN PLAY WITH THE GLYCAEMIC INDEX?

INSULIN IS A HORMONE PRODUCED by the pancreas and its role is to store away glucose from the bloodstream that isn't immediately needed for energy.

The increase in blood glucose levels after eating prompts the body to release insulin. When high-GI foods are eaten, the rapid increase in blood glucose causes a surge of insulin to be produced and this rapidly stores away the glucose that is circulating in the bloodstream.

You're probably familiar with this feeling – a 'high' feeling after eating a sugary food followed by a 'crash' as the glucose leaves your bloodstream. This is why one biscuit is never enough! Your body is trying to find a balance between the sugar high and the subsequent low by craving yet more sugar. Simply by doing its job, insulin is part of the cycle that causes food – and specifically, sugar cravings.

So how can we break out of this cycle? The answer is to avoid those very high-GI, sugary foods in the first place! As we know, low- and medium-GI foods lead to a much more gradual rise in blood glucose levels. This means they also prompt a much more sedate insulin response and when we eat primarily lower GI foods, we don't experience the same sugar highs and crashing lows as when we eat high-GI foods. By avoiding high-GI foods, we don't take that first ride on the blood glucose/insulin roller-coaster!

as glucose. Instead, fructose is transported to the liver where is it metabolized. Only then is it released as glucose, or it can be stored in the liver as glycogen. So fructose owes its lower GI value to the fact that is it taken out of circulation and is metabolized in a different way from other sugars. You'll see fructose available commercially in supermarkets along with the other sugars and sweeteners.

Artificial sweeteners have lower GI values still. Lactitol, for example, has a GI value of just 2 while xylitol, the sweetener found in many sweets and chewing gums, has a GI value of 7–8. Swapping ordinary sugar for a smaller amount of fructose or artificial sweetener in cooking makes an easy low GI swap.

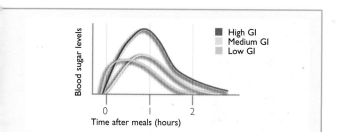

Think about your breakfast. If you start the day with high-GI corn flakes or puffed rice, for example, you are starting your day with a sugar rush, closely followed by an insulin rush, closely followed by a sugar low. You'll soon be hungry again and the foods your body will be craving are the high-GI foods that got you into trouble in the first place.

Start your day with low-GI 100% bran or medium-GI porridge instead. The energy from these foods is released much more gradually. You've avoided a peak in blood glucose and so you've also avoided a peak in insulin production. You'll feel fuller for longer so you won't get the same kind of food cravings and you certainly won't be as tempted to clear the biscuit trolley come mid-morning!

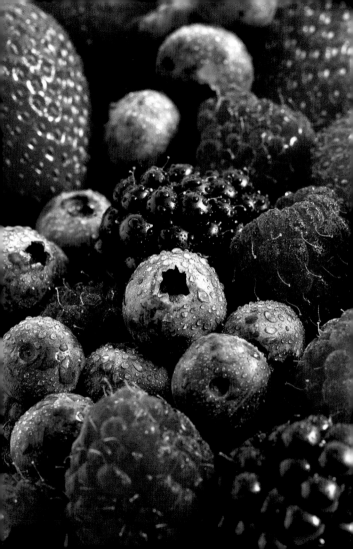

putting GI principles into practice

How do I recognize low-GI foods?

As we've seen, the glycaemic index is a method of ranking carbohydrate foods based on their effect on blood glucose levels.

Unfortunately, the GI value of a food isn't something we can generally read off food labels or work out using the nutrition information, although many supermarkets and some food manufacturers are beginning to show the GI categories on foods they have tested.

We need to find food GI values in lists or tables, such as the one at the back of this book (see pages 118–143), but there are rules of thumb that can help us make lower GI decisions.

♥ the more refined a food is, the higher the GI

Take bread, for example. Wholegrain bread is a medium-GI food with values generally ranging from 48 to 65. White bread is made with flour that has been stripped of its outer husk, lowering its nutrient and fibre content. This brings it into the high GI category with values ranging between 70 and 100.

So choose wholegrain foods over 'white' or refined versions whenever possible: go for wholegrain bread instead of white and use wholemeal flour instead of white flour, choose brown rice instead of white and select higher fibre breakfast cereals.

♥ the more processing a food has undergone, the higher the GI

Processing means that a food is easier for your body to break down – you don't need to do as much work to get at the nutrition. So if we make it easier on the body, we raise the GI of the food.

NO!	**YES!**
✖ cornflakes	✓ porridge or muesli
✖ watermelon	✓ berries
✖ white sliced ham sandwich	✓ ham sandwich with granary bread or wholemeal pitta
✖ chocolate chip cookies	✓ dark chocolate or a handful of M&Ms
✖ baked potato	✓ new potatoes
✖ curry with white rice	✓ fresh tagliatelle with vegetables

Boiled new potatoes, still in their skins, are medium GI (around 57). But if we choose instant mashed potatoes that have been processed in the factory, then we're choosing a high-GI food (values range from 74 to 97).

Think about processing that you do yourself at home as well as processing carried out by food manufacturers. When we drink the juice we have squeezed from fruit, we are throwing away fibre that is useful for lowering GI values and so are generally taking a higher GI food than if we ate the whole fruit.

Even cooking can raise the GI of food. Raw carrots, for example, have a low GI value of just 16 but when these are cooked, the carbohydrates become more easily available to the body and so have a much higher GI value of around 50.

♥ protein and fat lower the GI of a carbohydrate-rich food

Blood sugar levels are only influenced rapidly by the carbohydrate in food so protein and fat cannot be given GI values – they have theoretical GI values of 0. So carbohydrate foods that are also sources of protein and/or fat tend to have lower GI values.

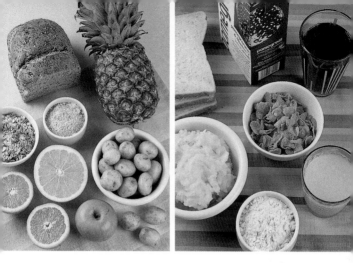

▲ *Whole foods tend to have lower GI values than their refined counterparts, so choose fruit over fruit juice, boiled new potatoes instead of mash and wholegrain, not white, carbohydrates.*

Take legumes – lentils, peas and beans. These are classed as carbohydrate foods but are rich sources of protein as well as fibre and this combination of nutrients serves to lower their GI. Legumes generally have GI values around the 30-mark.

This makes foods that are based on, or contain, legumes good low GI choices. Hummus, dhal, lentil soup and bean chilli, for example, are all good lower GI choices.

Fat has the same effect on food – it can lower the GI of carbohydrate-based foods. But remember, this means it will also increase the calorie content so we need to be careful about how much of it we eat.

Nuts have low GI values (ranging from 7 to around 22) thanks to their high fat content. In the case of nuts, the fat they provide

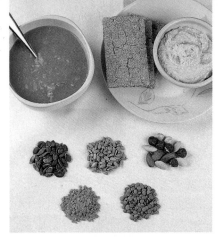

◀ *Beans are rich in protein and fibre, while nuts also provide fat, so these carbohydrate-rich foods have low GI values.*

is healthy poly- and mono-unsaturated fat but they are still extremely calorie-dense. So while they are low GI options, their calorie content means they aren't great choices for anyone trying to lose weight.

♥ combine higher GI foods with lower GI foods to lower the overall GI of a meal

One of the great things about following the principles of GI is that it gives you the freedom to include just about every food in your diet! A key point to remember is that the GI of a meal containing high-GI foods can be lowered by the inclusion of lower GI foods.

Baked potatoes fall into the high GI category. But top your potato with low GI baked beans and you have a medium-GI meal. Make low GI hummus or a small amount of peanut butter your favourite topping for high GI rice cakes, and you have a medium-GI snack. By being smart about combining foods, you don't have to take anything off the menu!

Combining high- and low-GI foods

Combining low-GI with high-GI foods lowers the overall GI of a meal, which means that practically no foods are off limits! The following examples all amount to medium-GI meals.

HIGH GI	+	LOW GI
cornflakes	+	All-bran
rice cakes	+	peanut butter
dates	+	sultanas and mixed nuts
slice of baguette	+	hummus
baked potato	+	reduced sugar baked beans
slice of watermelon	+	selection of fruit including berries, orange, kiwi and peach

= MEDIUM GI

♥ choose foods that are lower in sugar!

A simple rule to bear in mind is to choose foods that are less sweet. This doesn't only mean popping sugar-free muesli and reduced-sugar baked beans into your trolley, but also eating the bananas in the fruit bowl before they get too ripe. Yes, over-ripe bananas have a higher GI value than those that are slightly under-ripe!

▶ *Go for foods with less sugar – reduced sugar versions of tinned goods, breakfast cereals and even less ripe fruit.*

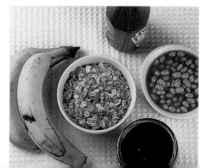

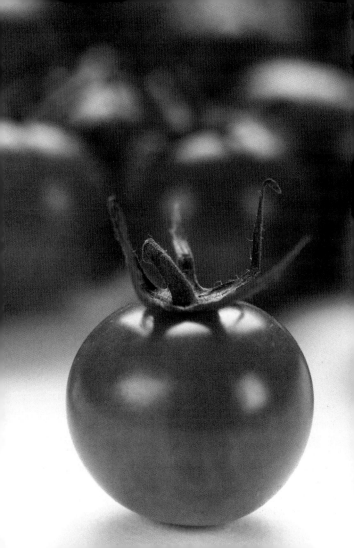

what will GI do for me?

Have you ever tried following a new diet plan only to feel absolutely exhausted by the end of day one? This certainly isn't going to happen when you follow the principles of low GI eating – and this is why we can follow this style of eating for life. Just some of the benefits you can expect are:

♥ avoiding energy highs and lows

If you're fed up with feeling drained and lacking in energy by mid-morning, then you need to follow GI!

Because low-GI foods release their energy slowly and gradually, your own energy levels will be much more stable. Think back to our blood glucose roller-coaster: high-GI foods give a quick sugar boost and give you that sugar 'high' feeling followed all too soon by a crash, as insulin does its thing and stores that blood glucose away in adipose (fat) tissue. When you eat low GI, you avoid those highs and lows, instead having more sustained energy levels.

Whether you're running around after the children all day, need to get through the working day or want to run a marathon, you'll feel the benefit of having more get-up-and-go!

♥ feeling fuller for longer

When you choose low GI carbohydrate foods over high GI versions, you will naturally increase the fibre intake in your diet. A slice of wholegrain bread has 2.1 g of dietary fibre, while a slice of white bread has only 0.5 g. Fibre adds bulk to foods, giving a feeling of satiety or fullness. And since it can't be digested by the body, it stays in the digestive tract for longer, making that satiated feeling last so much longer.

♥ avoiding food cravings

Imagine not needing to visit the vending machine mid-morning or not wanting to raid the biscuit tin in the evening! When you avoid high-GI foods, you avoid the blood glucose highs that accompany them and you also skip out the lows that occur when all that sugar is stored away.

It's those lows that make us crave more sugary foods – your body is simply trying to regain some kind of balance. But eat low GI and your body won't be thrown off-balance in the first place and you avoid those overwhelming food cravings that drive you to the cookie jar!

♥ lowering your risk

Regularly eating high-GI foods means that the body is continually having to produce the hormone insulin to deal with all the sugar. Over time, this means that we gradually need to produce more and more insulin for it to have the same effects on our bodies – this is known as insulin resistance. Impaired sensitivity to insulin can leave us vulnerable to metabolic syndrome or pre-diabetes (see box on page 31) and to diabetes.

Low-GI diets are also associated with higher HDL cholesterol levels – that's the healthy type of cholesterol that can help lower our risk of heart disease. And high fibre intake, which is more closely linked with low rather than high GI diets, can lower cholesterol, reduce the risk of heart disease and is associated with a lower risk of developing many forms of cancer.

GI and weight loss

There are thousands of different diets around and you might have tried one of them or you might have tried 20 of them over the years. Some of these diets do have a solid basis in science, some are just ridiculous but one thing most of them have in common

IS GI SUITABLE FOR THE WHOLE FAMILY?

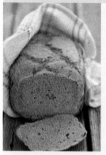

WHO WANTS TO COME HOME from a long day at work and cook two meals — one for you and one for the rest of the family? If you've followed diet plans in the past, you've probably done just that. But busy lives don't leave us time to run a restaurant in our kitchens every night, so for healthy eating to fit into our lives, it has to meet the dietary needs of all the family members.

It's not recommended for children to follow weight-loss plans. But GI isn't a weight-loss plan. Yes, it can make weight loss easier, but it's also a way to improve eating habits, even for those who aren't worried about their weight. And that includes kids.

Healthy eating is important for everyone and your decision to eat low GI could have a positive impact on your child's dietary habits. Parents are their children's greatest role models. If your kids see you choosing wholegrain bread instead of white or swapping your biscuit snack for a banana, they are likely to do the same — eventually! And if you don't put biscuits and chocolate bars in the trolley any more, the whole family will be the healthier for it!

Children under 10 years of age shouldn't be given low-fat or 'diet' products. They need energy from healthy sources and it's better that they get that energy from wholegrain cereal with full-fat milk than chocolate bars and fizzy drinks!

is that they require you to make sweeping changes to the way you usually eat. So, for the duration of the diet, you eat only foods beginning with the letter 'A' or have a grapefruit with every meal, and at the end of the diet, you go back to the unhealthy eating habits that made you gain weight in the first place. You gain back the weight – often with a little more, and go on another diet. And so the cycle continues...

Why should GI be any different?

Well, for a start, let's define the word 'diet'. Look this up in a dictionary and you'll find it's described as 'the food we *usually* eat'. So for any weight-loss diet to be successful, it has to reflect the food you *usually* eat. If a 'diet' calls for extraordinary changes to your eating habits, say, in what or when you have to eat, you won't be able to maintain that diet and it's only natural you should fall off the wagon. Cue disappointment and frustration.

GI is different. Following the principles of GI *can* fit into your life. You don't need to make a radical overhaul to your life to accommodate these principles, never eating out again or only ever shopping in health food stores. GI can work for you simply through making small decisions when you choose a meal from a menu, walk around the supermarket or cook the evening meal.

To lose weight, we need to take in fewer calories than we burn. GI makes it easier for us to take in fewer calories in two ways:

♥ the foods that have lower values on the glycaemic index are more filling and satisfying than foods that have higher values

♥ by avoiding high-GI foods, we avoid riding the blood sugar roller-coaster that makes us crave sugary foods and stimulates appetite.

Following GI principles is not a magic bullet to weight loss – portion sizes still matter and calories still count – but enjoying filling and satisfying low-GI foods makes it much easier for us to feel comfortable eating less food.

GI and diabetes

The glycaemic index was first developed as a way to help those with diabetes choose healthier carbohydrate foods and calculate carbohydrate exchanges.

There are two forms of diabetes: type 1 is an autoimmune disease in which insulin cannot be made and must be injected. Type 2 diabetes can develop when the body becomes less sensitive to insulin or cannot produce enough insulin to cope with the sugar being ingested. Type 2 diabetes used to be called 'adult-onset' diabetes because it was only seen in adults, but it is becoming more common to see type 2 diabetes in children, as we become heavier and less active as a nation.

GI AND METABOLIC SYNDROME

METABOLIC SYNDROME, SYNDROME X or pre-diabetes is a relatively recently recognized disorder of insulin metabolism. It is thought that metabolic syndrome increases an individual's risk of diabetes and/or cardiovascular disease.

There has been much controversy and debate about metabolic syndrome, even over the existence of the condition, but the International Diabetes Federation (IDF) recently defined metabolic syndrome as abdominal obesity plus high triglycerides, or high cholesterol, or high blood pressure, or high blood glucose levels.

How can GI help?

The continual production of insulin in response to high-GI foods means that the body gradually becomes de-sensitized to insulin, so the body has to produce more insulin to have the same effect. Following the principles of low GI eating means this situation won't occur and the body's insulin response won't be compromised.

Constant insulin production also promotes the creation of adipose tissue, or fat cells, especially around the abdomen. An apple body shape pre-disposes an individual to metabolic syndrome and diabetes (see page 149).

Low-GI diets tend to be higher in fibre which are associated with lower cholesterol levels. Following GI principles also helps stabilize blood glucose levels and can help lower the risk of developing type 2 diabetes.

GI is useful for the whole population but it is especially helpful for those with diabetes. Avoiding high-GI carbohydrates helps those with diabetes avoid peaks in blood sugar levels, making it easier to manage medications and avoid hypoglycemic episodes.

If close relatives have diabetes, your own risk is increased. But following the principles of GI can help you lower that risk. Low-GI foods don't prompt sudden surges of insulin so we can remain sensitive to the insulin that is produced. It's whenever we become de-sensitized to insulin and our bodies need to make more and more to cope with dietary carbohydrates that type 2 diabetes can develop.

How is low GI different to low carb?

Over the past few years, we've seen an unprecedented peak in the popularity of low-carb diets. While this may be on the wane, what makes low GI a winning proposition?

As their name suggests, low-carb diets all but exclude carbohydrates from the diet. Carbohydrate intake can be as little as 20 g per day, although it is recommended that these 20 g come from low-carb vegetables. At later stages, foods such as fruit and wholegrain bread can be re-introduced.

GI is different because it does not recommend excluding this valuable food group from the diet to the extent that low-carb diets do. It doesn't recommend excluding carbs at all! It recommends being smart with the carbohydrates you eat.

Out go the empty calories from sweets and fizzy drinks. Out go the foods that are so easily broken down that they cause our bodies to produce surges of insulin. Instead, we focus on healthy carbohydrate foods that provide us with fibre, nutrients and the body's preferred source of energy.

While low-carb diets can be difficult to follow, GI can fit easily into your lifestyle. Where low carb flies in the face of traditional healthy eating advice, low GI can be used to complement trusted guidelines. And while there is still controversy over the long-term safety of low-carb diets, there are no known down-sides to following low GI principles.

Is low fat dead?

If there is one criticism of low GI it is that low GI diets could potentially be high-fat diets. We've seen that both protein and fat-based foods cannot have their GI values tested because it is only carbohydrates that affect blood glucose levels. So a high fat content can lower the GI value of a food.

If you look at GI food tables (see pages 118–143), you might be surprised by some of the categorizations. Sponge cake, ice-cream,

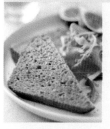

WHERE DOES PROTEIN FIT IN?

WHEN IT COMES TO FILLING YOUR PLATE, be sure to add some protein in there, too!

We know that we should be choosing lower GI carbohydrates, foods that are moderate in total fat (and as low as possible in saturated and trans fats), but what about that other macronutrient, protein?

Protein is an important addition to our healthy eating plate, not only because it has a number of jobs to do in the body, but also because protein has a high satiety value. That means it makes us feel full and satisfied. A sandwich filled with tuna or ham is more satisfying than a sandwich filled with the same caloric value of tomatoes, say.

As protein is also often linked with fat, it's important to choose protein foods wisely. Go for lean cuts of meat, remove the skin from poultry, swap meat for plant proteins every so often, enjoying legumes, tofu and nuts.

chocolate nut spread and chocolate are all low- or medium-GI foods. The addition of peanut butter brings high GI white bread down into the medium-GI category.

It's the fat content of these foods that lowers their GI. So does this means we can eat all the ice-cream and chocolate nut spread we fancy and still be eating healthily? Sorry, no. If we want to eat a healthy diet, balance is key. By all means, enjoy peanut butter on your wholegrain toast but remember that peanut butter is still an energy-dense food and will still provide plenty of calories and fat.

The healthiest food choices are those that are low on the glycaemic index, low in saturated and trans fats (these are the processed fats labelled as 'hydrogenated fats' on ingredient lists) and are nutrient-dense, that is, they provide plenty of nutrients for the number of calories they provide. Think of it as greater nutritional bang for your buck!

Good carb + good fat = good health

So, what's the recipe for healthy eating? Low GI carbohydrates, unsaturated fats and lean protein sources are all important inclusions in our daily diet. Add these to at least five servings of fruit and vegetables every day and three to four servings of dairy (or equivalent), and you have the recipe for healthy eating!

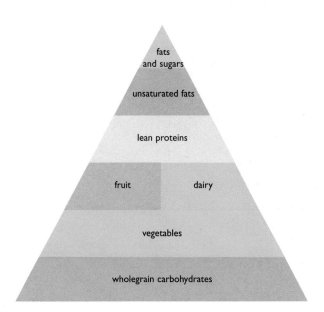

▲ The food pyramid shows us how much of the different food groups we should be eating: we should eat plenty of wholegrain carbohydrates and vegetables but very little fat and sugar.

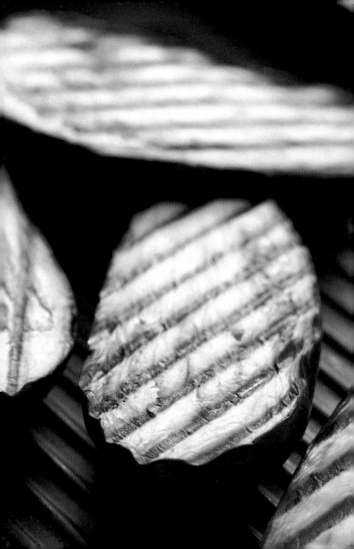

smart shopping

Being clever about your shopping basket is your first step to eating low GI. If you have plenty of healthy low- and medium-GI foods available in the larder, fridge and freezer, then it's only natural that these will form the basis of your meals. Keep high-GI foods to a minimum and the balance of your diet will certainly fall into the lower end of the GI scale.

In this chapter, we're going to categorize many common foods you might put into your shopping basket into 'often', 'sometimes' and 'rarely'. These categories reflect how often you should buy and eat these foods based not only on their GI value but on their overall value in a healthy diet.

For example, chocolate nut spread has a low GI value but since it is high in fat and calories, this will be placed in the 'sometimes' category. Watermelon has a high GI value but is a valuable food in the diet as it is a low-calorie, low-fat food rich in vitamins and minerals. This will also be found in the 'sometimes' category.

Foods that have low GI values and are low in fat will be in the 'often' category, while foods that are higher on the glycaemic index and high in fat, or otherwise have little nutritional value, will be found in the 'rarely' category.

It's important to remember that while GI is extremely useful in helping us choose healthy carbohydrate foods, other factors still apply. When we're trying to lose weight, portion size and calories still count, we should still try to limit our fat, especially saturated fat, intake and keep an eye on salt levels.

Tables showing foods categorized by GI value alone can be found at the back of this book (see pages 118–143). So, let's take a shop-by-shop look at your new basket!

Grocer

One of the simplest ways to ensure your shopping trolley is a healthy one is to shop mostly around the perimeter of the supermarket. If this sounds like an unusual piece of advice, think about how your local store is laid out – fruit and vegetables are presented just as you walk in, bread, meat, dairy and frozen foods are probably around or near the walls of the store, and the inside aisles are taken over with biscuits, cakes, crisps and fizzy drinks. These are the aisles to avoid! So, what's hot and what's not at the supermarket?

PACKAGE GOODS	OFTEN	SOMETIMES	RARELY
BISCUITS		crackers and crispbread	chocolate biscuits
		oat biscuits	digestives
		rice cakes	shortbread
		rich tea	
BREAKFAST CEREAL	100% bran	Fruit 'n' Fibre	bran flakes
	porridge	granola	Cheerios
	oat cereal	instant porridge	corn flakes
		muesli	Rice Crispies
		Special K	Pop Tarts
		sultana or raisin bran	Shredded Wheat
		wheat biscuits	sugar-, chocolate- and honey-coated cereal

PACKAGE GOODS	OFTEN	SOMETIMES	RARELY
BAKING INGREDIENTS	artificial sweeteners dried fruit gram flour wholemeal flour	mincemeat plain, milk and white chocolate	cake mix cornflour solid animal or vegetable fats icing sugar (any type) white flour
CONFECTIONERY	liquorice sugar-free chewing gum	muesli bar nougat peanut M&Ms plain, milk and white chocolate	chocolate bars jelly beans
CRISPS AND SNACKS	dried fruit	nuts pretzels rice cakes	breadsticks crisps popcorn
COOKING SAUCES	black or yellow bean sauces chilli sauce piri piri sauce tomato-, pepper and olive-based pasta sauces tomato-based curry sauce	barbecue cooking sauce honey mustard sauce nut-based sauce, such as satay sweet and sour stir-fry sauce wine-based cooking sauces	butter sauces, such as Hollandaise coconut- or cream-based curry sauces

PACKAGE GOODS	OFTEN	SOMETIMES	RARELY
FATS AND OILS	olive oil	olive oil margarine rapeseed or flaxseed oil nut oils wheatgerm oil vegetable oils and margarines	animal fats, such as butter and lard coconut oil hydrogenated canola oil vegetable oil solid vegetable fat or shortening
PICKLES, PRESERVES AND SPREADS	chutney pickles vinegar	chocolate nut spread honey peanut butter reduced sugar jam and marmalade	syrup treacle
PASTA, RICE AND OTHER FILLERS	barley bulgar wheat pasta wild rice	basmati rice brown rice couscous polenta quinoa rice noodles soba noodles	arborio rice croutons instant mashed potatoes instant noodles sticky rice stuffing white rice

PACKAGE GOODS	OFTEN	SOMETIMES	RARELY
SAUCES, FLAVOURINGS AND DRESSINGS	fat-free salad dressing herbs mustard soy sauce (reduced sodium versions) spices tomato-based salsa	pesto reduced fat mayonnaise salad dressing tartar sauce tomato ketchup	flavouring mixes high in sugar and salt mayonnaise
TINNED FOODS	fruit in juice lower fat milk puddings lentil or bean-based soups reduced salt and sugar baked beans vegetable soup vegetables (no added sugar or salt)	meat or poultry in sauce pasta meals	cream soups fruit in syrup fruit pie filling

DRINKS	OFTEN	SOMETIMES	RARELY
COLD DRINKS	fruit and low-fat dairy smoothies flavoured (zero calorie) water no added sugar cordial water	flavoured milk (low-fat versions) no added sugar fizzy drinks and mixers pure fruit juice vitamin-fortified cordials	energy drinks (after exercise only) fruit juice drinks full sugar fizzy drinks full sugar cordials
HOT DRINKS	de-caffeinated tea and coffee herbal and fruit teas low fat / low calorie / diet chocolate drinks	caffeinated tea and coffee cocoa low fat malted drinks	chocolate drinks (full fat, full sugar) malted drinks (full fat, full sugar)

FROZEN FOODS	OFTEN	SOMETIMES	RARELY
FROZEN FISH PRODUCTS	whole fish or fish pieces	breaded and battered white fish (oven-baked) fishcakes fish fingers fish in low-fat sauce	breaded and battered white fish (deep-fried) fish pie (pastry or potato-topped)

FROZEN FOODS	OFTEN	SOMETIMES	RARELY
FROZEN VEGETABLES	quick-frozen vegetables	root vegetables stir-fry vegetables sweetcorn vegetables in sauce	battered or breaded vegetables, such as onions or mushrooms mashed carrot and swede roasting parsnips
FROZEN POTATOES AND CHIPS		oven chips	roasting potatoes flavoured wedges flavoured oven chips frying potato chips mashed potato potato waffles and fritters
FROZEN READY MEALS	steam-cuisine style meals, especially those with new potatoes, noodles, chicken or fish	*meals with:* basmati rice brown rice noodles pasta tomato- or vegetable-based sauce	crispy pancakes hot pots *meals with:* cream, cheese or coconut-based sauces dumplings mashed potato jasmine rice pilau rice Yorkshire puddings

FROZEN FOODS	OFTEN	SOMETIMES	RARELY
FROZEN PIZZA AND BREADS		thin crust pizza with vegetables, chicken or lean ham margherita wholegrain garlic bread	processed meat, extra cheese toppings pizza pie thick crust stuffed crust white garlic baguettes
FROZEN MEAT AND POULTRY PRODUCTS	chicken breast fillets chicken fillet strips	100% beef burgers, grilled pork burgers turkey burgers	beef burgers, grillsteaks and ribsteaks breaded and battered chicken or turkey chicken Kiev sausages
FROZEN DESSERTS AND ICE CREAM		Pavlova and other meringue desserts frozen yoghurt reduced fat / sugar ice cream sorbet summer pudding and other fruit desserts	cakes and gateaux cheesecake pies and pastries premium ice cream

Greengrocer

It is recommended that we eat at least five portions of fruit and vegetables every day – two pieces of fruit and three servings of vegetables. All fruit and vegetables are healthy additions to your diet. However, when you want to follow low GI principles, then some are better choices than others.

FOODS	OFTEN	SOMETIMES	RARELY
FRUIT	all other fruit	over-ripe bananas watermelon	banana chips dried fruit coated in oil glacé fruit fruit canned in syrup
HERBS AND SPICES	all other fresh and dried herbs and spices		oil-based curry paste salt-based seasonings
POTTED SALADS	bean salad fruit and nut rice lentil salad pasta salad tabbouleh	couscous salad Florida salad reduced-fat coleslaw wild, basmati or brown rice-based salad	cheese coleslaw coleslaw (full fat, full sugar) white rice-based salad potato salad

FOODS	OFTEN	SOMETIMES	RARELY
SALADS	all salad vegetables		Caesar salad bacon bits/lardons full-fat dressing croutons
VEGETABLES	all other vegetables	carrots, cooked new potatoes boiled, in skins other root vegetables, mashed or roasted sweet potatoes	parsnips potatoes (baked, chipped, mashed, roasted)

Butcher

We've seen that protein-based foods, such as meat, fish and poultry, cannot have their GI value tested since they contain little or no carbohydrate. But there are still good and not-so-good choices to be found in the butcher, based on fat content and processing.

MEAT	OFTEN	SOMETIMES	RARELY
BEEF		lean beef	fatty cuts of beef, such as mince
LAMB		lean lamb	
PORK, BACON AND GAMMON	pork tenderloin	pork chops ham gammon	bacon
POULTRY	white meat	dark meat	poultry skin
GAME		all lean game	
SAUSAGES AND BURGERS		reduced fat or extra lean sausages and burgers	all other sausages and burgers
COOKED MEATS	chicken and turkey breast slices	lean ham pastrami	salami and other spicy sausage
VEGETARIAN AND MEAT ALTERNATIVES	Quorn tofu	vegetable burgers and fingers	

Fishmonger

Most of us don't eat enough fish! We're recommended to eat fish three to four times a week, with two of those portions being oily fish. An exception is made here for pregnant women, who should only eat oily fish once weekly due to potential mercury contamination in oily fish.

FOODS	OFTEN	SOMETIMES	RARELY
FISH	oily fish (2–3 times weekly) shellfish white fish	breaded and battered white fish (oven-baked) fishcakes fish fingers fish in low-fat sauce	breaded and battered white fish (deep-fried) fish pie (pastry- or potato-topped)

Bakery

Making smart GI choices is vital when visiting the bakery! High GI breads, hidden – and not-so-hidden – sugars lurk on every shelf and many of the goods on offer will have been made with refined flour, stripped of all its goodness.

FOODS	OFTEN	SOMETIMES	RARELY
BREAD AND ROLLS		granary, multi-grain and wholegrain bread and rolls	baguette white bread and rolls
MORNING GOODS		fruit loaf malt loaf	bagel croissant English muffin pancakes
ETHNIC BREADS	pumpernickel wholegrain pitta bread	tortilla white pitta bread	flatbread taco shells (fried) naan poppadom
CAKES		wholegrain/oat muffins	all other cakes
PASTRIES			all pastries and doughnuts

Health food store

Is everything in a health food store healthy? Despite the name, not everything on sale in a health food store is necessarily a healthy or low GI choice. Reading nutrition labels is vital here as there might be some GI pitfalls to avoid.

FOODS	OFTEN	SOMETIMES	RARELY
DRIED FRUIT	all other dried fruit	dried fruit coated in oil	fruit in chocolate or yoghurt coating
NUTS	all other nuts	chocolate-covered nuts yoghurt-covered nuts	oil-roasted nuts salted nuts
SEEDS	all other seeds		oil-roasted seeds

Dairy

Being rich sources of protein and fat, dairy products are relatively low in carbs and the carbohydrate they do contain is primarily lactose, which is a low GI sugar (values range from 43 to 48). Get smart with dairy by choosing lower fat versions.

FOODS	OFTEN	SOMETIMES	RARELY
BUTTER AND MARGARINE	low-fat vegetable spread reduced-fat olive margarine	full-fat olive and vegetable spreads	butter solid animal and vegetable fat hydrogenated vegetable oil
MILK	skimmed and semi-skimmed milk	flavoured skimmed milk drinks	full-fat milk Jersey milk breakfast milk
CREAM		reduced fat crème fraîche	all other cream
CHEESE	cottage cheese extra-light cream cheese	cheese spread light cream cheese naturally lower fat cheese, such as Edam or Gouda	full-fat blue cheese full-fat cream cheese reduced-fat hard cheese full-fat hard cheese full-fat soft cheese

FOODS	OFTEN	SOMETIMES	RARELY
EGGS		eggs	
YOGHURT	low-fat fruit yoghurt low-fat fromage frais low-fat natural yoghurt low-fat yoghurt drinks reduced-fat Greek-style yoghurt	full-fat Greek-style yoghurt full-fat natural yoghurt	custard-style yoghurt full-fat fruit flavour yoghurt 'luxury' yoghurt yoghurt 'corners'
DESSERTS	reduced fat milk desserts, such as custard and rice pudding	reduced fat fruit or chocolate mousse	full-fat milk desserts full-fat fruit or chocolate mousse 'twinpot' desserts

Ready-prepared foods

In this time-poor age, many of us rely on ready meals and pre-prepared foods to help us get dinner on the table in the evening. These foods can be a life-saver from time to time but it's important to remember that the processing these foods undergo depletes their nutrient value, generally increases their fat content and raises their GI.

FOODS	OFTEN	SOMETIMES	RARELY
READY MEALS	steam-cuisine style meals, especially those with new potatoes, noodles, chicken or fish	*meals with:* basmati rice brown rice noodles pasta tomato or vegetable-based sauces	crispy pancakes hot pots *meals with:* cream, cheese or coconut-based sauces dumplings mashed potato jasmine rice pilau rice Yorkshire puddings
PIZZA AND BREAD		thin crust pizza with vegetables, chicken or lean ham margherita wholegrain garlic bread	processed meat extra cheese toppings pizza pie thick crust stuffed crust white garlic baguettes

FOODS	OFTEN	SOMETIMES	RARELY
PIES, PASTRIES AND SLICES			all pastry pies and slices potato-topped pie
PORK PIE, SAUSAGE ROLLS AND SCOTCH EGGS			all pork pies, Scotch eggs and sausage rolls
QUICHE		reduced-fat vegetable quiche	all other quiche and egg-based flans
FRESH PASTA AND SAUCES	fresh pasta tomato-based sauces, such as arrabiata and napolitana	cheese or meat-filled pasta pesto	cheese or cream-based sauces, such as carbonara four-cheese, mushroom or mascarpone
FRESH SOUP	bean or lentil soup noodle soup soup with pasta vegetable soup vegetable and meat broth	soup with rice	cream soups parsnip soup soup with cheese, such as broccoli and Stilton

FOODS	OFTEN	SOMETIMES	RARELY
SANDWICHES AND SUSHI	all other sushi *sandwich fillings:* avocado beans (any type) chicken lean ham or beef lower fat cheese prawns tuna salmon	bread: granary, multi-grain, wholegrain *sandwich fillings:* full-fat cheese peanut butter	sushi with sticky rice bread: white *sandwich fillings:* bacon full-fat egg mayonnaise full-fat mayonnaise sausage
PARTY FOOD	smoked salmon crudités tomato-based salsa	low-fat dairy dips chicken skewers mini pakora and samosas	cocktail sausages full-fat dips mini Scotch eggs mini spring rolls mini pizzas sausage rolls

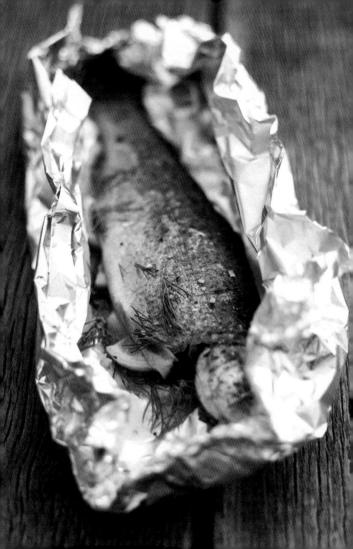

cooking methods matter...

So, now you have lots of lovely healthy foods in the fridge, what are you going to do with them? Cooking methods matter. How you decide to cook your food can change it from being a healthy food to an unhealthy food or can help transform a relatively unhealthy choice from a 'no-go' food to a 'once in a while' food. Just look at the difference cooking methods can make to the humble potato:

• medium-sized baked potato (175g): 161 cals and 0.2 g fat
• equal sized portion of potato mashed with milk and butter: 195cals and 7.3 g fat
• equal sized portion of French fries: 537 cals and 27.6 g fat

Healthy cooking methods

Method	What's so good about it?	What's not so great?	What can I cook?
STEAMING	– since food doesn't come into contact with water, all vitamins are retained – no fat is added	– not suitable for meat – doesn't add flavour	– dim sum – fish – new potatoes in their skins – some kinds of bread – vegetables
BOILING	– easy way to cook vegetables – no fat is added	– it's easy to overcook, losing water-soluble vitamins and colour – can cause loss of flavour and texture, especially through overcooking	– legumes – potatoes – vegetables

Healthy cooking methods

Method	What's so good about it?	What's not so great?	What can I cook?
STIR-FRYING	– quick method which retains flavour and texture of food – uses very little fat – one-pot meal so cuts down on the washing up!	– all foods need to be prepared in advance – cooking so fast at such high temperatures can be scary for the beginner!	– meat, fish and poultry – noodle and rice dishes – vegetables
MICROWAVE	– super-quick way to cook – uses very little water so vitamins in vegetables are retained – versatile – no saucepans to wash!	– texture, especially of vegetables, can become chewy, not crisp	– meat, fish and poultry – rice – stewed fruit – vegetables
GRILLING	– helps dry out fat from meat, fish and poultry – enhances colour and flavour through caramelization – marinades can add extra flavour and moisture	– can dry food out, especially if overcooked	– meat, fish and poultry – vegetables, such as tomatoes, aubergines and courgettes
BBQ	– allows excess fat to drip away – enhances flavour and colour – marinades can add extra flavour and moisture	– unreliable method, it's easy to over- and undercook food	– meat, fish and poultry – vegetables, such as tomatoes, aubergines, corn on the cob, courgettes, potatoes

Unhealthy cooking methods

Method	What's so good about it?	What's not so great?	What can I cook?
FRYING	– suitable for a wide range of foods – quick	– adds fat, doesn't allow fat already in food to drain away	– bread and potatoes – eggs – meat, fish and poultry
DEEP-FRYING	– quick – gives a crisp texture	– adds fat, doesn't allow fat already in food to drain away – requires specialist equipment; deep-frying in a pan can be dangerous	– meat, fish and poultry – vegetables

Neither here nor there...

Method	What's so good about it?	What's not so great?	What can I cook?
ROASTING	– enhances flavour, texture and colour – allows fat to drain, for example, in meats	– adds fat, for example, in vegetables	– meat, fish and poultry – vegetables
GRIDDLING	– enhances flavour, texture and colour – the pan ridges allow fat to drain, for example, in meats – relatively quick	– adds fat, for example, in vegetables	– meat, fish and poultry – vegetables

USEFUL KITCHEN EQUIPMENT

Sharp knives

Good knives will make things quicker and safer in the kitchen. Good basics are: 8-inch cook's knife, bread knife, serrated multi-purpose knife, paring knife

Grater

Texture can add variety: grate courgettes and cook as a rosti to replace plain old boiled slices. Grating can also make food such as cheese go further so you can use less.

Micro-whisk

Very handy to have around when cooking eggs, making sauces or muffins.

Fat-straining jug

Pour meat juices or stock into this jug, let the excess fat rise to the surface and drain off the healthier stock!

Selection of chopping boards

Try to keep specific chopping boards for specific purposes with separate boards for raw meat, fish and poultry, cooked meat, fish and poultry, and other ingredients.

Spray for oil

Cut down on the fat you add to food with an oil spray.

Immersion blender

Make soup-making a whizz!

Roasting rack

Place meat for roasting on a rack instead of straight into the roasting tin, and allow excess fat to drain away. Pour the juices through the fat-straining jug for a healthier gravy, too.

Steamer

You don't need to invest in
an electric steamer, unless
you plan to steam entire
meals on a regular basis.
Use a steamer saucepan
instead or simply place food
in a sieve or colander over
a pan of boiling water.

Bread machine

Baking your own bread gives
you control over what goes
into it. Use wholegrain
flours, add seeds, cut down
on sugar – these will all give
a healthier loaf. Of course,
bread can still be made by
hand but a machine makes
bread-making a lot easier.

Slow cooker

In this time-poor age, there's
nothing nicer than coming
home to find dinner ready!
Pop the ingredients into the
cooker in the morning, turn
it on and then go about your
day – dinner will be ready
4 to 8 hours later. Also a
great way to make stock –
cover the carcass from a
roast chicken with water,
add onions, celery and
herbs, and simply leave
to cook slowly for 8 to 10
hours.

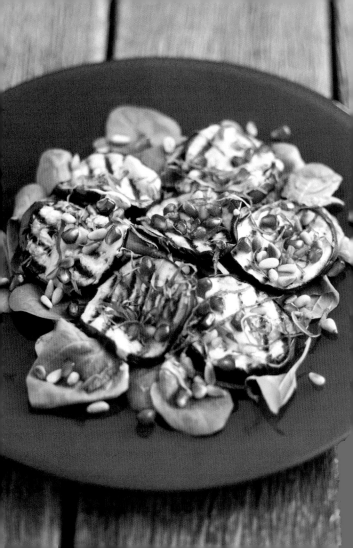

what can I eat?

Eating the low GI way

If you look back to Chapter 4, you'll see the foods that you should be buying often, sometimes and rarely. The foods in the 'often' category are those that you should base your diet around. These are the low-GI and low-fat foods that make up the basis of a healthy diet. This doesn't mean that you need to shun the rest of the foods. A healthy diet, and especially a diet that follows the principles of the glycaemic index, is about balance.

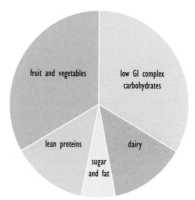

Let's think about the healthy eating plate. The healthy eating plate is an easy way to tell if your meals follow healthy eating principles. The main points to bear in mind are:

♥ one third of your plate should be made up of fruit and vegetables

♥ another third should be low GI complex carbohydrates

♥ the final third should be split between lean proteins, dairy products and sources of sugar and fat

When it comes to making good GI choices here, bear these rules in mind:

Vegetables

♥ fruit and vegetables are the key to healthy eating. We should all be aiming to eat *at least* three portions of vegetables and two portions of fruit every day (see box below)

♥ try to limit high GI vegetables such as parsnips and cooked carrots as much as possible. Now, when we're told to avoid something, that

---

WHAT IS A PORTION?

A FRUIT OR VEGETABLE PORTION is equivalent to 80 g or any of these:

I apple, banana, pear, orange or other similar sized fruit
2 plums or similar sized fruit
1/2 a grapefruit or avocado
I slice of large fruit, such as melon or pineapple
3 heaped tablespoons of vegetables (raw, cooked, frozen or tinned)
3 heaped tablespoons of beans and pulses (however much you eat, beans and pulses count as a maximum of one portion a day)
3 heaped tablespoons of fruit salad (fresh or tinned in fruit juice) or stewed fruit
I heaped tablespoon of dried fruit (such as raisins and apricots)
I cupful of grapes, cherries or berries
I dessert bowl of salad
I glass (150 ml) of fruit juice (however much you drink, fruit juice counts as a maximum of one portion a day)

GLYCAEMIC LOAD

ANOTHER CONCEPT TO THINK ABOUT IS that of glycaemic load. Glycaemic load, or GL, is calculated as the GI of a food multiplied by the amount of carbohydrate in that food divided by 100.

GL is useful because it gives another way to gauge the impact of different foods to the body in terms of how much carbohydrate they provide. So GL gives us information on the amount of carbohydrate in a food in relation to its GI. In a similar way to GI, GL levels are split into low, medium and high categories:

Low GL =10 or below

Medium GL = 11–19

High GL = 20 or above

Let's look at a few examples to illustrate how useful GL can be. We know that parsnips have high a GI value of 97. If we look at the nutritional content of parsnips, we find that they provide 12 g carbohydrate in every 100 g food. To work out their GL we perform the following calculation:

97 x 12 / 100 = 11.6

So parsnips have a medium GL. In practice, this means that, although their carbohydrate structure gives them a high GI value, the actual amount of carbohydrate in parsnips means that they only have a medium impact on the body.

Watermelon also has a high GI value of 72. With 6.8 g carbohydrate per 100 g food, their GL works out as 4.9 – a low GL value. So while the carbs in watermelon are the types of carbs that are broken down quickly and produce a high GI value, there aren't enough of them to illicit a high glycaemic response. Watermelon is, after all, mostly water so there just aren't enough of these high GI carbs in your slice of watermelon to cause a major impact on the body.

Finally, let's look at a low–GI food – dark chocolate. It has a low GI value (34) but each 100 g chocolate provides 57 g carbohydrate, so its GL is calculated to be 19.4. The types of carbohydrates in dark chocolate (together with its high fat content) have a low impact on the body in terms of GI. However, there are so many of these carbohydrates that, overall, a piece of chocolate has a much greater glycaemic impact on the body than the foods which have high GI values but low carbohydrate content.

often makes it all the more attractive. So instead of focusing on what you can't have, think of all the fabulous fruit and veg you *can* have! There are so many delicious low GI vegetables around that you will be spoilt for choice! Buttered asparagus, griddled aubergine, hearty bean casseroles, spiced cauliflower, crisp mange-touts, roast onions, baked tomatoes... the choices are endless!

♥ when choosing fruit, go for the lower GI options. This means the only fruit you need to think about limiting are melon and tropical fruit, such as papaya, pineapple and over-ripe bananas. But it's important to remember that fruit – all fruit – are still healthy foods. This is where a concept known as glycaemic load comes in (see page 65).

Complex carbohydrates

♥ choose primarily low GI carbohydrates and keep medium– and high-GI carbs to a minimum. This might mean swapping sticky rice for brown or basmati rice, having boiled new potatoes instead of mash or choosing rye bread instead of refined white bread.

Proteins

♥ protein has a high satiety value, that is, it helps us feel full, so include a lean protein food at every meal. Poultry (without skin), fish and lean cuts of red meat are healthier choices than processed meats like sausages or bacon, or high-fat mince and the like. Remember that plant protein counts too, so have beans, nuts, seeds or soy foods several times a week instead of red meat.

Dairy

♥ dairy foods are our main source of calcium, needed to keep bones and teeth strong. Full-fat dairy foods do provide a lot of animal fat, however, so always go for lower fat options – skimmed or semi-skimmed milk, lower fat yoghurt and lower fat cheese.

Sugars

♥ sugary foods provide empty calories – that is, they provide energy without any nutrients. Processed sugary foods are also notoriously high-GI foods so these are the foods you want to limit more than any others. Biscuits, sweets, cakes and sugary drinks add no goodness at all to your diet.

Fats

♥ fats have high energy density in that they have lots of calories in relation to the nutrition they provide. But, unlike sugars, fats also have functions and so we need small amounts of these in our diets. It's important, though, to be smart about what fats are included. Saturated and trans fats harm our bodies, raising cholesterol, clogging arteries and promoting free radical damage. Unsaturated fats, however, actively protect the body, lower cholesterol, are used in brain and nerve development and help hormone balance. So limit animal and processed fats and choose instead plant fats and oils from olives, nuts, seeds, avocados and sunflowers.

FOOD GROUP	ENJOY THESE...	... INSTEAD OF THESE
FRUIT	apples berries citrus fruit stone fruit	melon over-ripe bananas pineapple papaya

VEGETABLES	aubergines
	beans, peas and legumes
	carrots (raw)
	courgettes
	cruciferous vegetables,
	  such as broccoli,
	  cauliflower and sprouts
	leafy greens
	mushrooms
	peppers
	tomatoes
		broad beans
		carrots (cooked)
		parsnips

COMPLEX CARBOHYDRATES	basmati, brown and wild rice new potatoes pasta white rice sweet potatoes	gnocchi mashed potatoes white bread
PROTEINS	fish lean red meat poultry (without skin)	fatty red meat

DAIRY	fromage frais
	lower fat cheese
	lower fat yoghurt
	skimmed and semi-
	  skimmed milk
		full-fat dairy
		sour cream and
		  full fat crème fraîche

FOOD GROUP	ENJOY THESE...	... INSTEAD OF THESE
SUGARS	fructose honey maple syrup	other sugars processed sugary foods like biscuits, sweets and fizzy drinks
FATS	avocado nuts and seeds and their oils olives olive oil vegetable oil	fatty red meat, processed meat products full–fat dairy hard animal fat, lard or dripping hard vegetable shortening poultry with skin on

GI: FINDING YOUR BALANCE

ONE OF THE GREAT THINGS ABOUT GI is that high- and low-GI foods can balance each other.

Think of it like a see-saw with high-GI foods on one side and low-GI foods on the other: these effectively cancel each other out and when we eat low- and high-GI foods together, we actually eat a medium-GI meal.

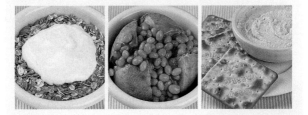

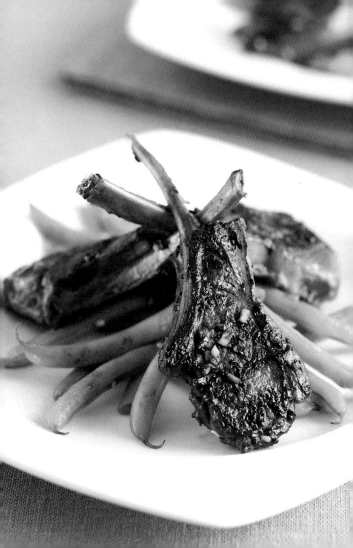

GI: meal-by-meal

Breakfast: the most important meal of the day

You've heard the old saying a million times before – breakfast like a king, lunch like a prince and dine like a pauper. Well, it's true. Breakfast is the most important meal of the day, and here's why.

When you sleep, your metabolic rate – the rate at which your body burns calories – slows down. And your metabolic rate will stay slowed down until you eat again. Breakfast means just that – you are breaking your overnight fast. So, if you eat at 7 am, your body will move up a gear and will burn calories more efficiently from then on. If you don't eat until noon, however, your body has spent five extra hours in slow-motion – time when your body has been saving, not using, energy most efficiently.

But it's not only important to eat breakfast – it's important to eat the right breakfast. Start the day with high GI cereal and you've stepped right on the roller-coaster. You'll probably feel hungry again pretty quickly and because your body is trying to balance its blood sugars, you might well be craving more refined, GI carbs fairly soon. That explains the mid-morning biscuit break.

Swap that high GI cereal for a lower GI muesli, cereal or porridge and you start the day with a steady and gradual rise in blood sugars. There will be no more energy highs and lows and you'll be much less tempted by the tea trolley.

So, what are the best and worst breakfast choices? Keep these foods in your larder and you'll always have the means to prepare a healthy breakfast:

Store-cupboard stand-bys

Carbohydrate foods
porridge oats
lower sugar muesli
high fibre bran cereal, such as 100% bran
wholegrain bread
rye bread or pumpernickel
wholegrain, low sugar muffins

Protein foods
cottage cheese
high protein snack bars
eggs

Fats
reduced-fat olive margarine
reduced-fat vegetable margarine

Dairy
semi-skimmed and skimmed milk
lower fat yoghurt
probiotic drinks
dairy smoothies

Fruit and vegetables
fruit, especially apples, berries, citrus fruit, pears and
 stone fruit
dried fruit, preferably without oil
fruit smoothies
unsweetened fruit juice

Top 10 best breakfasts

1 sugar-free muesli with nuts, topped with natural low-fat yoghurt
2 porridge with dried fruit, such as prunes or figs
3 fruit and yoghurt smoothie
4 medium-GI cereal, such as bran flakes or malt flakes topped with 100% bran, with semi-skimmed milk
5 boiled egg with wholegrain toast, spread with reduced-fat olive margarine, and an orange
6 reduced sugar and salt baked beans with granary toast
7 peanut butter and banana on wholegrain toast
8 pumpernickel with cheese or ham and a glass of unsweetened fruit juice
9 mixed berries with yoghurt
10 high protein, low sugar, high fibre breakfast bar

Top 10 worst breakfasts

1 high GI cereal, such as corn flakes or puffed rice with full-fat milk and sugar
2 traditional fry-up
3 white toast with butter and full-sugar jam or marmalade
4 white flour pancakes with syrup
5 sausage rolls
6 white flour bagels
7 full sugar, low protein, low fibre cereal bars
8 muffins
9 croissants and pain au chocolat
10 no breakfast!

Lunch: your mid-day top up

Did you know that the average lunch hour is actually only about 27 minutes? More and more of us are eating at our desks, eating on the go or eating nothing at all. And while breakfast is vital to kick-start the metabolism in the morning, each meal of the day plays its own role in keeping the body ticking over. Eating often means that blood sugars are kept stable and we avoid the highs and lows of fluctuating energy. Eating little and often also means that we avoid ever getting too hungry – so hungry that we grab whatever's going, no matter how unhealthy it might be!

A good lunch will help you avoid energy crashes and make it all the easier for you to resist the lure of the tea trolley mid after-noon! Low GI carb choices and lean protein combined with fruit and vegetable portions add up to a healthy and satisfying lunch.

Store-cupboard stand-bys

Carbohydrate foods
wholegrain bread and rolls
pumpernickel
pitta bread
flour tortillas
rye crispbread
pasta
basmati and brown rice
quinoa
reduced salt and sugar baked beans
legumes
barley
bulgar (cracked wheat)

Store-cupboard stand-bys

Protein foods
roast chicken
lean ham
tuna and salmon, canned in brine
lower fat cheese
lentil and bean soup
lentil or bean salad

Fats
reduced–fat olive margarine
reduced-fat vegetable margarine
olive oil

Dairy
lower fat cheese
lower fat yoghurt
dairy smoothies

Fruit and vegetables
salad and vegetables
vegetable soup (not cream versions)
fruit, especially apples, berries, citrus fruit, pears and
stone fruit
fruit smoothies
unsweetened fruit juice

Top 10 best packed lunches

1 tuna mixed with celery, diced peppers and a little natural yoghurt, with salad and a wholegrain roll
2 pasta salad with beans and feta cheese
3 pumpernickel with lower fat cheese, fruit
4 chicken, tomato salsa and salad in a wholegrain tortilla
5 mixed beans with diced sweet potato in pitta
6 chicken and avocado wrap
7 basmati rice, lentil and nut salad
8 Greek salad
9 pitta with cottage cheese, cherry tomatoes and rocket
10 hummus on rye crispbread, fruit and fromage frais

Top 10 best cooked lunches

1 reduced salt and sugar baked beans on granary toast
2 stir–fry with noodles, vegetables and crushed cashew nuts
3 minestrone soup, stewed apple with low–fat custard
4 ham and asparagus omelette
5 warm spinach salad with cherry tomatoes and grilled bacon
6 poached eggs with grilled tomatoes and wholegrain toast
7 grilled mature cheese on wholegrain toast with a side salad
8 new potato salad with salmon
9 chicken noodle soup
10 turkey rashers with wholegrain bread

Top 10 worst lunches

1 baked potato with cheese
2 pie or pasty
3 burger in white bun
4 bacon or sausage in a white roll
5 full-fat cheese on baguette
6 pâté on white melba toast
7 stuffing in a sandwich
8 extra cheese or meat thick-crust/stuffed-crust pizza
9 fried eggs with fried bread or potato waffles
10 creamy soup

Dinner: keep up the good work!

For many of us, the evening meal is the main meal of the day. It's also a chance to wind down, catch up with family and friends and relax.

Ending the day on a high GI meal doesn't pose quite the same concerns as a high GI breakfast does – since you'll be going to bed soon, there isn't the same potential for a full day of energy highs and lows. However, eat a high GI meal in the evening and you might find yourself snacking in front of the TV or even unable to sleep because too much sugar leaves you feeling uncomfortable.

If you enjoy a glass of wine, with dinner is the time to have it. Have a drink before dinner and your blood sugars will dip, stimulating appetite and possibly making you less conscious of the food choices you're making. So have your wine with your meal and the impact of alcohol on blood sugars is lessened.

Store-cupboard stand-bys

Carbohydrate foods
pasta
basmati or brown rice
new potatoes
quinoa
flour tortillas
bulgar (cracked wheat)
barley
legumes
reduced salt and sugar baked beans
sweet potatoes

Store-cupboard stand-bys

Protein foods

chicken or turkey,
 without skin
white and oily fish
lean pork
lean beef or lamb
legumes
lentil or bean soup
nuts and seeds

Fats

olive oil
rapeseed (canola) oil
nut oils

Dairy

lower fat cheese
small amounts of strongly
 flavoured cheese
lower fat crème fraîche
Greek and low-fat natural
 yoghurt
fromage frais

Fruit and vegetables

aubergines
beans
courgettes
cruciferous vegetables,
 such as broccoli,
 cauliflower and sprouts
leafy greens
legumes
mushrooms
peas
peppers
raw carrots
tomatoes
salad vegetables
sweet potatoes
vegetable soup
 (not cream versions)
fruit, especially apples,
 berries, citrus fruit, pears
 and stone fruit

Top 10 best dinners

1 pasta with salmon and broccoli
2 baked chicken in spiced yoghurt with brown rice
3 grilled steak with new potatoes
4 bean fajitas
5 chickpea and sweet potato curry
6 steamed cod with roast tomatoes
7 green lentil soup
8 noodles with tofu, stir–fried vegetables and cashew nuts
9 omelette or fritatta
10 lamb casserole with cannellini beans

Top 10 worst dinners

1 pizza with garlic bread
2 baked potatoes with sour cream dip
3 fried sausages with mashed potatoes
4 pastry-topped pie
5 burgers and hot dogs
6 sticky rice sushi
7 gnocchi
8 risotto
9 creamy or coconut curry with naan bread or jasmine rice
10 dumplings and stuffing

Snacks: little and often to boost energy

When following the principles of low GI eating, it's a good idea to eat little and often. So instead of basing your daily intake around three main meals, think instead about having a greater number of mini meals. By all means, still eat at breakfast time, lunchtime and in the evening, but eat in between, too.

Snacking has traditionally been frowned upon as an unhealthy habit but what makes snacks unhealthy are the food choices. As well as choosing sugary and fatty snacks, we have often consumed these in addition to our three main meals.

The key to healthy snacking is to choose healthier options and to view these as part of your overall daily diet. Snacks mid-morning and mid–afternoon can help keep blood sugars – and energy levels – stable. Avoid getting too hungry and you also avoid the risk of making less healthy food choices because you're starving or have to resort to the vending machine.

So, depending on when you eat your main meals, you might like to have a snack in the middle of the morning. If you eat a late evening meal, one or two snacks will easily fit into your afternoon, or if you eat an early dinner, you might prefer one snack mid-afternoon and another supper-time snack.

What you snack on might also depend on where you are at the time. It's not very convenient to try spreading hummus on crackers when you're standing on the train but this is a great snack if you're still at your desk or at home when you snack. For the commute, keep fruit or cereal bars in your bag and take a yoghurt drink from the fridge just as you set out.

If you decide to snack, you do need to adjust your main meals accordingly so your energy or fat intake doesn't soar. Keep snacks handy – in your desk drawer, in the car or in your handbag so you're always in control of what you eat.

Store-cupboard stand-bys

Carbohydrate foods

wholegrain bread and rolls
lower sugar muesli
high fibre bran cereal,
 such as 100% bran
wholegrain bread
rye bread or pumpernickel
crispbread
wholegrain, low sugar
 muffins

Protein foods

high protein snack bars
cottage cheese
cheese sticks or triangles
nuts
seeds, such as pumpkin
 or sunflower

Fats

small amount of peanut
 butter
reduced–fat olive
 margarine
reduced–fat vegetable
 margarine
small amount of dark
 chocolate

Dairy

semi–skimmed and
 skimmed milk
lower fat yoghurt
probiotic drinks
dairy smoothies
yoghurt drinks

Fruit and vegetables

fruit, especially apples,
 berries, citrus fruit, pears
 and stone fruit
dried fruit, preferably
 without oil
unsweetened fruit juice
fruit smoothies
vegetable sticks, such as
 celery, peppers and
 carrots

Top 10 best snacks

1 small handful of mixed nuts
2 one piece of fruit
3 low–fat yoghurt with poppy & flaxseeds
4 veggie sticks with 2 Tbsp of hummus
5 banana and peanut butter on wholegrain toast
6 2 crispbread with 4 Tbsp of cottage cheese
7 couple of squares of dark chocolate
8 small bowl of sugar–free muesli with semi–skimmed milk
9 small handful of mixed dried fruit with pumpkin seeds
10 pot of lower fat custard

Top 10 worst snacks

1 chocolate bars
2 boiled or chewy sweets, such as jelly beans
3 sugary cereal bars
4 biscuits
5 cake
6 pastries
7 crisps
8 ice cream
9 high GI breakfast cereal, such as corn flakes with full–fat milk
10 tortilla chips

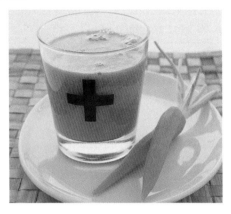

Drinks: don't drown your healthy diet!

So, we've now seen what makes the best and worst food choices. But what about drinks? Can a small glass of something really have that much of an impact on our diet?

Well, yes. Some drinks are pure sugar and will provide absolutely nothing other than calories. Other drinks will provide valuable nutrition in a low GI package so are obvious better choices. While a healthy and balanced diet does have room for the occasional drink in the former category, problems arise when these replace the nutritious drinks on a regular basis.

Just think about fizzy drinks. Children used to drink milk. Kids now drink fizzy drinks instead of milk. So not only are they adding sugar and empty calories, damaging teeth and increasing their intake of phosphates (linked to the leaching of calcium from bones) but they are losing out on a valuable source of calcium, fat–soluble vitamins and protein.

Beverage choices are as important as food choices. Here's what's what when it comes to drinks:

ENJOY

water: we should all aim to drinks 1 to 2 litres of water per day

flavoured (zero calorie) water, no added sugar cordial: the good news is, these will count towards your water quota for the day

fruit smoothies: fruit smoothies can count as one of your daily five fruit and veg portions and are a lower GI choice than fruit juice. This is because the whole fruit is used, including the fibre

low-fat dairy smoothies: these can count towards one of your three daily dairy servings

de-caffeinated tea or coffee: caffeine can cause blood sugars to drop so de-caff versions are a better option

herbal and fruit tea: these can also count towards your water quota. They can be a good source of antioxidants when green tea is included

low-fat malted drinks

low-fat/low-calorie chocolate drinks

MODERATE

flavoured milk (low-fat versions): these are great for kids but compare brands to find those with less sugar

no added sugar fizzy drinks and mixers: these don't provide the same 10 teaspoons of sugar that you'd find in a can of regular fizzy drink and can be a way to make the transition from fizzy pop to fizzy water

pure fruit juice: juice can count as one of your five fruit and vegetable portions per day but they are a concentrated sugar source

vitamin-fortified cordials: sugar-free cordial with vitamins would be your best choice of cordials

caffeinated tea or coffee

cocoa: this is also a caffeine source

LIMIT

energy drinks: these provide a rapid sugar hit and are suitable only when exercising

fruit juice drinks: fruit flavour drinks do not need to contain any actual fruit so will be pure sugar without the accompanying vitamins found in pure fruit juice

full-sugar cordials

full-sugar fizzy drinks: sugar, phosphate and acid, we're better off without!

full-fat, full-sugar chocolate drinks: these provide both sugar and fat so the lower calorie options are healthier choices

full-fat, full-sugar malted drinks

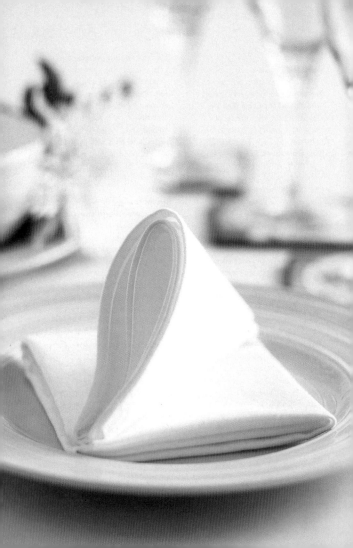

entertaining

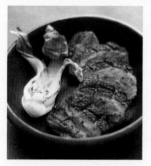

Entertaining at home is the perfect socializing solution for anyone worried about their diet. Not only do you get good company and an enjoyable evening – you also get total control over what you eat! And of course, healthy food doesn't have to be dull or mean. Eating healthily – and low GI – allows you to celebrate delicious food that has the added benefit of being good for you! Try any of these menu ideas next time you're throwing a dinner party.

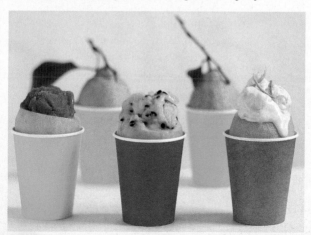

MENU I

Caprese-style salad

Alternate thick slices of ripe plum tomatoes with torn strips of buffalo mozzarella and wedges of avocado. Top with a few olives and lots of freshly torn basil. Drizzle with extra virgin olive oil just before serving.

Saltimbocca with roast new potatoes

Lay a slice of Parma ham on top of a thin escalop of veal (or flattened chicken fillet), top with a leaf of fresh sage and attach using a cocktail stick. Pan fry, then de-glaze the pan with Marsala wine and stir in a small knob of butter. Serve with par-boiled new potatoes finished off in a hot oven with extra virgin olive oil and freshly ground black pepper.

Strawberries with vanilla mascarpone

Mix together equal amounts of mascarpone cheese, natural low-fat yoghurt and Greek yoghurt. Stir in ½ tsp vanilla extract and serve with fresh strawberries.

MENU 2

Tom yam gung

Bring 750 ml (1½ pts) chicken stock to the boil and add 2 bruised stalks of lemongrass, 3 Tbsp nam pla, a 4–cm (1½-in) piece of sliced ginger, 6 lime leaves, juice of 1 lime and 4 sliced chillis. Add shelled and de-veined prawns and continue to simmer until the prawns are pink and cooked through. Add a bunch of chopped fresh coriander before serving.

Thai green chicken curry

Bring 400 ml (14 fl oz) reduced-fat coconut milk to the boil and add 2 tsp green curry paste. Add 450 g (1 lb) chicken cut into 2.5-cm (1-in) pieces, and simmer gently for 15 minutes, adding plenty of green vegetables, such as broccoli, green beans and pak choi in the last few minutes of cooking time.

Mango with lime

Mix the zest of 1 lime with ½ tsp fructose and a small bunch of chopped fresh mint; sprinkle over a plate of sliced mango.

MENU 3

Chicken liver pâté

Cook off 1 diced shallot, 200–300 g (7–10½ oz) chicken livers, torn fresh sage and a dessertspoonful of brandy. Blitz with a heaped dessertspoon of crème fraîche in the processor before serving, chilled, with toasted mixed grain baguette slices.

Roast beef with horseradish mash

Swap mashed potatoes for butter bean purée flavoured with horseradish sauce and serve with your favourite roast beef and green vegetables.

Rhubarb crumble

Add oats and nuts to your crumble topping and swap half the plain flour for wholegrain. This will turn a sugary fruit dessert into a valuable source of fibre, vitamins B and E and essential fatty acids.

MENU 4

Chicken skewers

Marinate chicken pieces in a mix of low-fat natural yoghurt, curry powder and a squeeze of lemon juice. Thread on skewers before cooking under a pre–heated grill or on a griddle pan.

Fish curry

Coat chunks of white fish 500 g (1 lb 2 oz) with $1/2$ tsp each ground coriander, cumin, turmeric and chilli powder. Set aside while softening 1 sliced onion with 2 crushed garlic cloves and 4 cm ($1\frac{1}{2}$ in) grated ginger. Add 2 diced tomatoes, 1 tsp tamarind paste dissolved in 100 ml (4 fl oz) water and 1 tsp creamed coconut and simmer for 10 minutes. Add the fish pieces and simmer for a further 10 mins. Serve with boiled basmati rice.

Pistachio ice cream

Time to cheat! Stir toasted pistachio nuts into good shop-bought ice cream and serve with tropical fruit salad.

MENU 5

Dips with vegetable and pitta sticks

 Serve homemade or shop-bought dips, such as hummus, baba ganoush, tzatziki and taramasalata with sticks of pepper, carrot and celery, and cauliflower and broccoli florets, as well as strips of toasted pitta bread.

Vegetable tagine with bulgar wheat

 Add a mixture of vegetable chunks, such as courgette, aubergine, sweet potatoes and tomatoes to softened onions and garlic. Season with cinnamon, cumin, ground coriander, oregano and harissa. Add a tin of drained and rinsed chickpeas and simmer for 30 minutes. Serve with bulgar wheat.

Poached figs

Melt 1 tsp honey into the juice of an orange, add 2 fresh figs per person to the pan and simmer very gently for 20 minutes. Top with sliced pistachio nuts or toasted sesame seeds and serve with low-fat Greek yoghurt.

MENU 6

Steamed asparagus

Steam asparagus spears for 4 minutes, then place in a small roasting tin, top with a mix of granary breadcrumbs, lemon zest and olive oil. Grill to brown before serving.

Salmon with roast vegetables

Combine 1 Tbsp each of chopped fresh basil, flat-leaf parsley, lemon juice and extra virgin olive oil and marinate salmon fillets for $\frac{1}{2}$ hour. Transfer to a baking tray and cook in a pre-heated oven, basting with the marinade for 10 minutes. Serve with roast vegetables and boiled new potatoes.

Summer pudding

Swap plain white bread in a summer pudding recipe for a mixed grain version and fill with ripe berries, sweetened with apple juice concentrate if necessary.

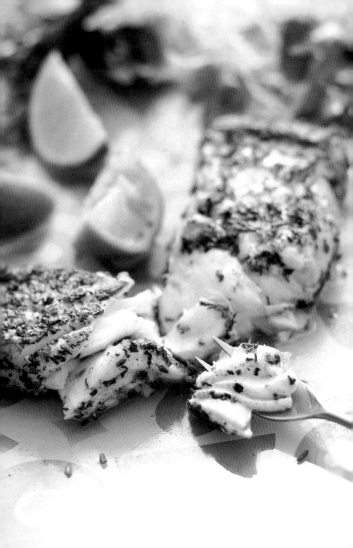

eating out

When we eat at home, we're in control of what we cook, how we cook it and how much we eat. But it's a different story when we go out to eat. Eating out is often a social occasion. We want to relax, enjoy ourselves and appreciate food that someone else has prepared for us.

It's been found that we eat significantly more when we eat with friends than if we eat alone. Interestingly, we also tend to eat more when we eat in front of the TV than when we eat at the table. This is really because our attention is distracted away from our food and towards the entertainment so we basically don't notice when we've eaten enough to satisfy our appetite.

The food on the menu could break every healthy eating guideline we usually follow but sound so tempting it's hard to say no. Or maybe we don't want to feel like a slave to healthy eating and instead want to push the boat out on a special occasion.

Even if we are still concerned with healthy options, there might not be too many on offer. And then portion sizes are a whole other matter!

Restaurant portions could often feed two. Since so many of us have been brought up as members of the 'clean plate club' we find it all but impossible not to finish everything on our plates, no matter when we stopped feeling hungry.

So how do we make smart choices when we're eating out, without feeling like martyrs to health? First, follow this survival guide and then use the examples over the coming pages to help you identify the good, the bad and the ugly on the menu.

TOP 10 TIPS FOR EATING OUT

1   Don't arrive hungry!

Arrive at a restaurant hungry and it's virtually impossible to make healthy choices. The secret is not to arrive so hungry that your self-control goes out the window! So, have a small bite to eat before you go out – this will keep your blood sugars stable so cravings don't take over when you read the menu. A piece of fruit, natural yoghurt or a small bowl of high fibre cereal are all ideal.

2   If possible, choose your meal ahead of time

Most restaurants will be happy to fax over their menu or they might have a website showing their current choices. When you've just finished your lunch or at some other time when you're not feeling hungry, take a look at their menu and decide in advance what you're going to have. Again, this will give you more control over making smart choices.

3   Drink water

Water is a great way to quell the hunger pangs so reach for the water jug, not the wine bottle, when you arrive. A big glass of water will take the edge off your hunger while a glass of wine, especially on an empty stomach, will cause your blood sugars to fall, making it doubly difficult to make smart choices.

4   Ask for the bread to be removed

Most restaurants will place a bread basket on the table when you arrive. The chances are this will be fluffy white bread – very tempting but you know it is nutritionally empty and the butter that's offered with it is just full of saturated fat. So move the basket out of reach or ask that it be removed, once your companions have taken what they wish.

5   Have a starter

A starter of soup or salad can help you eat less at your main meal. Go for a light, non creamy soup or a mixed green salad. Filling up with a starter will also make it that much easier to say 'no, thanks' when the sweet trolley comes around!

6   A bit on the side

Sauces and dressings are often full of fat or are thickened with white flour. So ask for any sauces to be served on the side so you can control how much you eat.

7   Lost in translation

Menus are often full of very tempting descriptions that are really just 'deep-fried' or 'full of sugar' in disguise. Crispy, coated, breaded, au gratin, creamy, cheesy, stuffed and caramelized are some terms to steer clear of.

8   Ask for what you want

The customer is always right! You are paying for your meal so ask if they can prepare your food how you like it, grilling instead of frying meat for example. Ask for details on side dishes, too, and ask for replacements if necessary – swap boiled white rice for brown, ask for new potatoes instead of chips or have extra vegetables instead of a starchy side-dish.

9   Ditch the dessert

Healthy desserts are thin on the ground but if you've had a starter, you're probably not going to still be hungry enough to really appreciate a sweet anyway. If you do like something sweet after a meal, go for fruit salad or order a more decadent dessert with plenty of forks so it can be shared around.

10   Be aware of drinks

Alcohol can cause fluctuations in blood sugars, making it less easy for you to control what and how much you eat and to recognize when you've eaten enough. Alcohol also adds empty calories. So if you are going to have a drink, make it a glass of red wine, which is a good source of powerful antioxidants, and have it when you're eating your meal as this will lessen the impact on blood sugars.

Round off a meal with de-caff coffee by all means but skip the sugar- and alcohol-laden liqueurs.

English

English food has a reputation for being heavy and stodgy. While there are certainly some healthy options available, much traditional English food is of the 'comfort' variety. Pies, mash, and fish and chips are just some of the not-so-healthy menu choices to steer clear of!

COURSE	YES PLEASE	JUST A LITTLE	NO THANKS
STARTERS	asparagus with a light vinaigrette avocado and crab salad fish: smoked salmon, prawns, sardines grilled mushrooms melon pâté: fish, vegetable, chicken vegetable-based soup	asparagus with Hollandaise sauce pâté: chicken liver or duck potato-based soups, such as leek and potato	cream or cheese soups pastry-based tart Welsh rarebit
MAINS	grilled or baked fish grilled or roast chicken new potatoes, boiled salads vegetables	braised lamb shank fishcakes game grilled or roast lean meat liver and bacon	bangers and mash cottage pie fish and chips mashed potatoes mushy peas pastry-topped pie

COURSE	YES PLEASE	JUST A LITTLE	NO THANKS
MAINS			ploughmans shepherd's pie steak and kidney pie toad in the hole
DESSERTS	fresh fruit lower fat custard stewed, baked or poached fruit	fruit crumble (wholegrain, oat or nutty topping) Pavlova sorbet summer pudding	bread and butter pudding chocolate brownies or cake fruit crumble (white flour topping) ice cream sponge puddings spotted dick trifle
DRINKS	de-caff tea or coffee herbal or fruit tea still or sparkling water	red or white wine	beer caffeinated drinks

Italian

The traditional Italian diet is extremely healthy – lean meat, poultry and plenty of fish accompanied by salads, fresh vegetables and olive oil. But somewhere along the way, we've come to think of Italian food as pasta smothered in a creamy sauce or pizza drowning in cheese and pepperoni. Let's get back to basics and look at the healthy and not so healthy choices in an Italian restaurant.

COURSE	YES PLEASE	JUST A LITTLE	NO THANKS
STARTERS	**fish:** calamari, clams, mussels, prawns, salmon (check this isn't fried) green or mixed salad minestrone soup olives vegetable antipasti zuppa di fagioli (bean soup) crostini	antipasti meats, such as bresaola and carpaccio bruschetta topped with beans or tomatoes	anti-pasti salami bread or breadsticks with dips breaded and deep-fried cheese bruschetta topped with cheese Caesar salad garlic bread, especially with extra mozzarella risotto
MAINS	baked, grilled or griddled fish baked, grilled or griddled lean poultry	lean grilled meat **meat sauces:** Bolognese pesto porchetta (pork)	breaded and fried chicken or **meat:** picatta dumplings gnocchi

COURSE	YES PLEASE	JUST A LITTLE	NO THANKS
MAINS	pasta, especially wholegrain *vegetable and tomato sauces:* arrabiata, napolitana, marinara, pomodoro, primavera, ragù with mushrooms salad vegetables	saltimbocca *wine sauces:* Marsala	*cheese sauces:* four-cheese, formaggio, mascarpone *creamy sauces:* alfredo, bechamel, carbonara, florentina mushroom sauce filled pasta lasagne meatballs risotto rosemary-roasted potatoes
DESSERTS	fresh fruit	fruit semi-freddo	gateaux tiramisù
DRINKS	de-caff tea or coffee herbal or fruit tea still or sparkling water	red or white wine	liqueurs, such as Amaretto Disaronno caffeinated drinks mocha

Pizza

Pizza isn't an innately healthy food, especially American-style deep-crust pizza, but damage limitation is possible!

COURSE	YES PLEASE	JUST A LITTLE	NO THANKS
STARTERS	salad	chicken wings (skin removed)	dips garlic bread ribs
MAINS	thin crust *toppings:* ham, chicken, Cajun chicken, tuna, chilli, mushrooms, onions, peppers, anchovies, tomatoes, olives, aubergine, capers, artichokes	thick crust *toppings:* beef, sweetcorn, pineapple	stuffed crust *toppings:* pepperoni, bacon, salami, sausage, meatballs, extra cheese
DESSERTS	fresh fruit	sorbet	cheesecake hot fudge sundae ice cream
DRINKS	de-caff tea or coffee fruit tea still or sparkling water	red or white wine	caffeinated herbal or drinks

American/Steakhouse

As well as making healthy choices, you'll need to keep an eye on portion sizes in American-style or steakhouse restaurants. Remember, the usual portion size for meat is around 100 g or 4 oz – not 24 oz!

COURSE	YES PLEASE	JUST A LITTLE	NO THANKS
STARTERS	*fish:* mussels, oysters, prawns, salmon (check these aren't fried) salad	vegetable-based soups chicken wings fish goujons shrimp cocktail	Caesar salad deep-fried stuffed mushrooms chicken goujons mozzarella sticks loaded potato skins onions rings ribs
MAINS	baked, grilled or griddled chicken fillet corn on the cob grilled or baked fish lean grilled pork salad vegetables	grilled lean burger grilled lean steak	baked potatoes battered and deep-fried meat, fish or poultry cheeseburger fries hash browns onion rings ribs white burger buns
DESSERTS	fresh fruit	sorbet	apple pie cheesecake hot fudge sundae pecan pie
DRINKS	de-caff tea or coffee herbal or fruit tea still or sparkling water	red or white wine	caffeinated drinks

Chinese

Traditional Chinese food can be very healthy but many restaurants now feature deep-fried dishes and sugary sauces that mean we need to be careful about what we choose.

COURSE	YES PLEASE	JUST A LITTLE	NO THANKS

STARTERS	chicken and sweetcorn soup
	crab soup
	hot and sour soup
	lettuce wraps:
	  chicken or vegetarian
	  shredded chicken
		chicken skewers
		lettuce wraps with
		  mince meat
		wonton soup
			chicken balls
			crispy duck with
			  pancakes
			crispy seaweed
			deep-fried
			  spring rolls
			deep-fried
			  wontons
			prawn crackers
			sesame toasts
			spare ribs

MAINS	black bean sauce
	fish: king prawns,
	  monkfish, sea bass,
	  scallops, sole,
	  squid
	stir-fried chicken
	  or pork
	  with vegetables
		boiled rice
		stir-fried beef or
		  duck with
		  vegetables
		chilli garlic sauce
		chow mein
		fried tofu
			battered and
			  deep-fried meat
			  or poultry
			'crispy' means
			deep-fried: crispy
			  beef, crispy'
			  noodles, etc.
			egg fried rice

COURSE	YES PLEASE	JUST A LITTLE	NO THANKS
MAINS	noodles steamed tofu *vegetables:* bamboo shoots, beansprouts, Chinese leaves, mushrooms, pak choi, spring onions, waterchestnuts yellow bean sauce	oyster sauce plum sauce sweet and sour sauce	'sizzling' means fried special fried rice sweet chilli sauce
DESSERTS	fresh fruit	lychees	fruit fritters toffee apples, bananas or pineapple
DRINKS	de-caff tea or coffee green, herbal, fruit or jasmine tea still or sparkling water	red or white wine	caffeinated drinks

Mexican

Mexican cooking uses a lot of beans – great news from both low GI and low-fat perspectives. But watch out for re-fried beans. Although these aren't actually fried, they are mashed, giving them a higher GI value. Many Mexican restaurants allow you to select your own ingredients to mix and match – this way you can skip unhealthier menu options like sour cream and fried corn taco shells.

COURSE	YES PLEASE	JUST A LITTLE	NO THANKS
STARTERS	bean soup fish: crab cakes mussels, salmon (check these aren't fried) gazpacho salad (without the extras like croutons or bacon)	habanero wings (skin removed) tortilla soup	Caesar salad nachos

COURSE	YES PLEASE	JUST A LITTLE	NO THANKS
MAINS	black beans baked, grilled or griddled chicken fillet chicken or shrimp salad * chicken or vegetable skewers flour tortilla garlic sauce grilled or baked fish or shellfish mole pepper salsa tomato salsa	grilled lean steak guacamole re-fried beans huevos rancheros huevos a la chimichangas mexicana corn tortillas	battered and deep-fried meat, fish or poultry sour cream white rice
DESSERTS	fresh fruit		
DRINKS	de-caff tea or coffee herbal or fruit tea still or sparkling water	red or white wine	caffeinated drinks tequila

Thai

Most Thai food is quite healthy, with plenty of lightly cooked vegetables, chicken and fish. Unhealthy options, however, are also to be found, and coconut milk is the main culprit. Coconut is the only nut that is full of unhealthy saturated fat so go for clear soups and curries that aren't based on coconut milk.

COURSE	YES PLEASE	JUST A LITTLE	NO THANKS
STARTERS	*clear soup:* tom yum gung, tom yum gai *noodle soup:* tom whusen musub *vegetable soup:* tom phak ruam fishcakes	*coconut soups:* tom kha gai, tom kha gung grilled satay skewers vegetable tempura	deep-fried chicken skewers spring rolls ribs deep-fried prawns

COURSE	YES PLEASE	JUST A LITTLE	NO THANKS
MAINS	stir-fried chicken or beef noodles fried rice	fried noodles fish with vegetables sweet and sour sauce noodle omelette pad thai	battered and or fried rice deep-fried meat, fish or poultry crispy duck (kao pad kai) jasmine or sticky rice (kao suey) meat, fish or poultry in coconut-based sauces, such as gaeng phet gai, gaeng kiew wan nua, guang kua supparod gung
DESSERTS	fresh fruit		
DRINKS	de-caff tea or coffee herbal or fruit tea still or sparkling water	red or white wine	caffeinated drinks

Fast food

Fast food used to mean a burger, fries and maybe another burger. Times have changed, thankfully, and there are healthier options in most fast-food restaurants. Salads and grilled sandwiches are among the healthier choices. Skipping toppings such as croutons will also make salads lower GI choices.

COURSE	YES PLEASE	JUST A LITTLE	NO THANKS
BREAKFAST	oatmeal	bagel with poly unsaturated margarine or light cream cheese	bacon, sausage and/or egg muffins bacon roll bagel with egg, bacon and cheese bagel with bacon, lettuce and tomato breakfast roll hash browns pancakes
BURGERS AND SANDWICHES	chicken sandwich (grilled) filled brown rolls, such as chicken salad, chicken tikka, sweet chilli chicken	filled brown rolls, such as cheese, ham and pepperoni, beef and cheese filled white rolls	burgers with bacon burgers with cheese burgers with more than one patty

COURSE	YES PLEASE	JUST A LITTLE	NO THANKS
BURGERS AND SANDWICHES	vegetable melt	fried fish sandwich hamburger grilled burgers grilled chicken baguettes veggie burger	fried chicken sandwich cheeseburger
SALADS	chicken salad with low-fat dressing garden salad with low-fat dressing	chicken salad with dressing and croutons crispy chicken salad	
SIDE ORDERS	carrot sticks	dips, such as BBQ or sweet and sour	French fries fried onion rings potato wedges
DESSERTS	fruit and yoghurt fruit bag	apple pie	doughnuts ice cream
DRINKS	de-caff tea or coffee herbal or fruit tea still or sparkling water milk orange juice	diet fizzy drinks	caffeinated drinks fizzy drinks milkshakes

French

The people of France tend to eat quite a rich diet, yet they have surprising low rates of heart disease. This "French Paradox" is thought to be down to the quantity of fresh fruit and vegetables, unsaturated oils and red wine included in the French diet. And while food is rich, portion sizes are small.

COURSE	YES PLEASE	JUST A LITTLE	NO THANKS
STARTERS	clear soup fruit lentil salad salade niçoise vegetable-based soup: onion *fish:* mussels, salmon	escargots (snails in butter)	pâté
MAINS	baked or grilled fish baked or grilled chicken fillet vegetables	lean beef	dauphinoise potatoes duck lamb
DESSERTS	fresh fruit	cheese	crème brûlée millefeuille tarte Tatin
DRINKS	de-caff tea or coffee herbal or fruit tea still or sparkling water	red or white wine	caffeinated drinks

Indian

Indian menus are awash with unhealthy choices but healthier options are there if you know what to look for – choosing tomato and vegetable–based sauces, chicken instead of red meat and noodles instead of pilau rice or naan bread will all keep your meal on the lighter side.

COURSE	YES PLEASE	JUST A LITTLE	NO THANKS
STARTERS	chicken skewers and kebabs (marinaded in yoghurt)		aloo tikka chat (fried potatoes) bhaji and samosas
MAINS	bhuna chutney dopiaza jalfrezi korai riata rogan josh tandoori	masala paneer	battered and deep-fried meat or poultry boiled rice butter chicken chapati ghee korma naan bread passanda pilau rice poppadom
DESSERTS	fresh fruit	kulfi	honey cakes
DRINKS	de-caff tea or coffee herbal or fruit tea still or sparkling water	chai red or white wine	caffeinated drinks

Mediterranean and Middle Eastern

The Mediterranean diet is one of the most healthy diets in the world. High intakes of fruit and vegetables, legumes and pulses, fish and nuts all combine to ensure that those eating a Mediterranean diet receive plenty of vitamins and minerals, unsaturated fats, anti-oxidants and fibre.

COURSE	YES PLEASE	JUST A LITTLE	NO THANKS
STARTERS	baba ganoush (aubergine dip)	*cured meats:* bresaola, Serrano ham	meatballs
			merguez (lamb sausages)
	fish: mussels, prawns (check these aren't fried)	falafels	saganaki (fried feta cheese)
	green salad	paella	
	harira (soup)	pissaladiere (vegetables and anchovy tart)	salami
	hummus		spanikopita and bourekas (spinach pastries)
	marinaded vegetables: artichokes, aubergine tomatoes, courgettes		
	zaaluk (roast vegetables)		

COURSE	YES PLEASE	JUST A LITTLE	NO THANKS
MAINS	caponata *kebabs:* chicken, fish fish green beans with almonds olives tabbouleh and bulgar wheat tagine vegetables ratatouille (vegetable stew)	couscous with vegetables, beans or chickpeas *kebabs:* beef, lamb, kefta rice–stuffed vine leaves	*tagine:* beef, lamb tzimmes (carrots with raisins and honey) bastilla (chicken filo pie) patatas bravas
DESSERTS	fresh fruit		baklava streusel
DRINKS	de-caff tea or coffee herbal or fruit tea still or sparkling water	red or white wine	caffeinated drinks

Japanese/Sushi

Sushi and sashimi are fundamentally healthy choices. But when you're following a low GI diet, choose dishes other than those with sushi rice – sticky rice has a very high GI of around 92.

COURSE	YES PLEASE	JUST A LITTLE	NO THANKS
STARTERS	edamama (steamed soy beans)	tempura	
MAINS	all other sushi and sashimi		*rice sushi:* California roll, norimaki, futo-maki mochi (rice cakes) *other rice dishes:* chakin-zushi, chirashi sushi, gohan senbei (rice crackers) dumplings
DESSERTS	fresh fruit		
DRINKS	de-caff tea or coffee green, herbal, fruit or jasmine tea still or sparkling water	red or white wine sake	caffeinated drinks

Vegetarian

Many people think that a vegetarian diet has to be healthier than one that includes meat – but this isn't necessarily so. Unhealthy options are still to be found! Vegetarians do need to be careful about their protein choices since protein is so often associated with fat.

COURSE	YES PLEASE	JUST A LITTLE	NO THANKS
STARTERS	guacamole		deep–fried cheese
	soup: vegetable, beans and lentil		
	sprouting salad		
MAINS	beans, peas and lentils	millet	battered or breaded deep-fried vegetables
	nuts		
	quinoa		
	quom		
	seeds		
	seitan		
	sweet potatoes		
	tempeh		
	tofu		
DESSERTS	fresh fruit	sorbet	
DRINKS	de-caff tea or coffee	red or white wine	caffeinated drinks
	herbal or fruit tea		
	still or sparkling water		

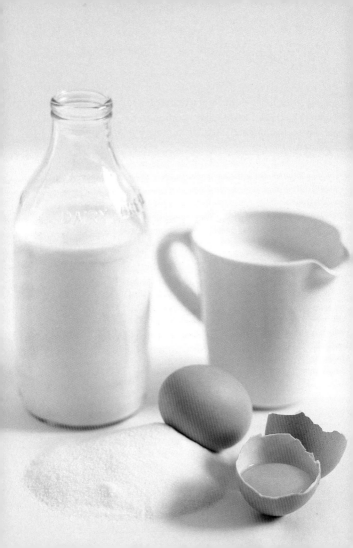

GI food tables

There are three tables in this chapter, showing foods divided into their GI categories of low, medium and high. We know that low-GI foods are not always the healthiest foods and that high-GI foods don't necessarily need to be avoided at all costs. For example, we've seen that fat content lowers the GI of foods so high-fat foods like red meat or butter actually have such low GI values that these can't even be tested. And some fruit have high GI values but aren't foods that we would want to cut out of our diets.

So in this chapter, we're dividing low-, medium- and high-GI foods into those that are healthy choices, unhealthy choices and those that are somewhere in between! These tables will give you all the information you need to make healthy, low-GI choices!

We've also seen that GI values are based on carbohydrate content. Some foods have so little carbohydrate that they just can't be tested. These are the foods that are high in protein, fat or just contain so much water that it wouldn't be possible to test their GI. These foods are designated as low GI but are marked with an asterisk (*) so you can distinguish these as naturally low carbohydrate foods.

Low GI (55 or below)

FOODS	HEALTHY CHOICES	ENJOY OCCASIONALLY	UNHEALTHIER CHOICES
CAKES		sponge cake	banana cake
			chocolate cake (from packed mix, with chocolate icing)
			madeira cake
			muffins: apple, chocolate, butterscotch
			vanilla cake (from packed mix, with vanilla icing)
BISCUITS	vita-wheat crackers	oat and honey	
		oatmeal	
		oatcakes	
		most plain chocolate biscuits	
		Rich Tea	

Low GI (55 or below)

FOODS	HEALTHY CHOICES	ENJOY OCCASIONALLY	UNHEALTHIER CHOICES
BREAD	barley bread		
	buckwheat bread		
	bulgar bread		
	fruit loaf		
	mixed grain bread		
	oat-bran bread		
	pumpernickel		
PASTA AND NOODLES	capellini	tortellini, cheese	
	fettuccine		
	gluten-free pasta		
	instant noodles		
	linguine		
	mung bean		
	noodles		
	macaroni		
	ravioli		
	rice noodles, fresh		
	spaghetti		

Low GI (55 or below)

FOODS	HEALTHY CHOICES	ENJOY OCCASIONALLY	UNHEALTHIER CHOICES
PASTA AND NOODLES	spirali		
	split pea and soy		
	pasta shells		
	vermicelli		
BREAKFAST CEREALS	100% bran		Frosties
	Alpen and other		
	muesli		
CEREALS	barley		
	bulgar		
	rye		
	sweetcorn		
PRESERVES AND SPREADS		marmalade	chocolate spread

Low GI (55 or below)

FOODS	HEALTHY CHOICES	ENJOY OCCASIONALLY	UNHEALTHIER CHOICES
CONFECTIONERY AND SNACKS		milk chocolate	Twix
		plain chocolate	
		white chocolate	
		peanut M&Ms	
		nougat	
LEGUMES	baked beans		
	blackeye beans		
	butter beans		
	chickpeas		
	green lentils		
	haricot beans		
	hummus		
	kidney beans		
	lima beans		
	marrowfat peas		
	mung beans		
	pigeon peas		
	pinto beans		

Low GI (55 or below)

FOODS	HEALTHY CHOICES	ENJOY OCCASIONALLY	UNHEALTHIER CHOICES
LEGUMES	romano beans		
	red lentils		
	soy beans		
	split yellow peas		
VEGETABLES	asparagus*		
	aubergine*		
	bamboo shoots*		
	beetroot greens*		
	broccoli*		
	cabbage (savoy, red, white*)		
	carrots (raw/cooked)		
	cauliflower*		
	celeriac*		
	celery*		
	chard*		
	courgettes*		
	cucumber*		

Low GI (55 or below)

FOODS	HEALTHY CHOICES	ENJOY OCCASIONALLY	UNHEALTHIER CHOICES
VEGETABLES	fennel*		
	garlic*		
	green beans*		
	lettuce*		
	mange-touts*		
	mushrooms*		
	okra*		
	olives*		
	onions*		
	pak choi*		
	peas		
	seaweed*		
	shallots*		
	spinach*		
	spring onions*		
	sprouts*		
	tomato*		
	turnip*		
	water chestnuts*		
	yam		

Low GI (55 or below)

FOODS	HEALTHY CHOICES	ENJOY OCCASIONALLY	UNHEALTHIER CHOICES
FRUIT	apples (fresh and dried)		
	avocado*		
	bananas		
	cherries		
	dried apricots		
	grapefruit		
	grapes		
	mango		
	oranges		
	peaches		
	pears (fresh and canned)		
	plums		
	strawberries		
FRUIT JUICE	apple juice, unsweetened		

Low GI (55 or below)

FOODS	HEALTHY CHOICES	ENJOY OCCASIONALLY	UNHEALTHIER CHOICES
FRUIT JUICE	apple and cherry juice		
	carrot juice		
	grapefruit juice, unsweetened		
	orange juice, unsweetened		
	pineapple juice, unsweetened		
	tomato juice, unsweetened		
MEAT	beef, lean*	cured meats, such as bresaola and pastrami*	bacon*
	offal*		beef, fatty (beefburger, mince, etc.)*
	pepperoni*		
	pork, lean*	ham*	
	veal*	lamb, lean*	lamb, fatty (mince, etc.)*

Low GI (55 or below)

FOODS	HEALTHY CHOICES	ENJOY OCCASIONALLY	UNHEALTHIER CHOICES
MEAT			pork, fatty (mince, etc.)* salami* sausages*
FISH	crab* lobster oily fish, such as herring, mackerel and salmon* shellfish, such as mussels, oysters and prawns* sushi white fish, such as cod, haddock, hoki plaice and sole*	breaded or battered fish* fish fingers	

Low GI (55 or below)

FOODS	HEALTHY CHOICES	ENJOY OCCASIONALLY	UNHEALTHIER CHOICES
POULTRY	chicken, white meat*	breaded or battered chicken*	chicken, skin*
	chicken breast slices*	chicken, dark meat*	turkey, skin*
	turkey, white meat*	turkey, dark meat*	
	turkey breast slices*		
	smoked turkey*		
	wafer-thin turkey slices*		
NUTS AND SEEDS		cashew nuts	
		peanuts	
		other nuts*	
		almond butter*	
		cashew butter*	
		peanut butter*	
		pumpkin seeds*	
		poppy seeds*	
		sesame seeds*	

Low GI (55 or below)

FOODS	HEALTHY CHOICES	ENJOY OCCASIONALLY	UNHEALTHIER CHOICES
NUTS AND SEEDS		sesame seed paste (tahini)* sunflower seeds*	
OTHER PROTEIN FOODS	eggs	high protein meal replacement bars	
DAIRY DESSERTS	reduced-fat custard	egg custard custard reduced-fat ice cream	premium ice cream reduced-fat mousse (commercial mix with water) instant pudding (chocolate or vanilla)
MILK AND NON-DAIRY ALTERNATIVES	skimmed milk soy milk	full-fat milk low-fat chocolate soy milk drinks	

Low GI (55 or below)

FOODS	HEALTHY CHOICES	ENJOY OCCASIONALLY	UNHEALTHIER CHOICES
YOGHURT AND NON-DAIRY ALTERNATIVES	fat-free yoghurt, with sweetener		
	reduced-fat yoghurt		
	yoghurt drink		
	soy yoghurt		
FATS AND OILS		avocado oil*	butter*
		cooking spray*	coconut oil*
		fish oil*	*dripping*
		groundnut oil*	ghee*
		nut oil*	hydrogenated
		olive oil*	vegetable oil*
		rapeseed (canola) oil	lard*
			palm
		safflower oil*	kernel oil*
		sesame oil*	palm oil*
		sunflower oil*	soy oil*
		vegetable oil*	*suet:* animal
		wheatgerm oil*	or vegetable*

Low GI (55 or below)

FOODS	HEALTHY CHOICES	ENJOY OCCASIONALLY	UNHEALTHIER CHOICES
DRINKS		banana soy smoothie	*sports drinks:*
			Sustagen Sport
		chocolate, hazelnut and soy smoothie	
		malt drinks	
		nutrient-fortified drinks	
		raspberry smoothie	
CONVENIENCE FOODS	sushi	chicken nuggets (baked)	chicken nuggets (fried)
	lentil soup	fish fingers	pizza, topped
	minestrone soup		sausages
	noodle soup		
	tarhana soup		
	tomato soup		

Medium GI (56–69)

FOODS	HEALTHY CHOICES	ENJOY OCCASIONALLY	UNHEALTHIER CHOICES
CAKES		angel food cake	flan cake
		muffins: apple,	
		oat and sultana,	
		apricot,	
		coconut and	
		honey, banana,	
		oat and honey,	
		bran, blueberry,	
		carrot, oatmeal	
BISCUITS	rye crispbread	arrowroot	
		digestives	
		cream crackers	
BREAD		crumpet	croissant
		fibre-enriched	hamburger bun
		white bread	Indian flatbread
		oat bread	pancakes
		spelt wheat bread	pastry

Medium GI (56–69)

FOODS	HEALTHY CHOICES	ENJOY OCCASIONALLY	UNHEALTHIER CHOICES
BREAD		sunflower and barley bread	pain au lait
			semolina bread
		wholemeal bread	sourdough
		white pitta bread	
PASTA AND NOODLES	rice noodles, dried and boiled	gnocchi	
	rice vermicelli		
	udon noodles		
BREAKFAST CEREALS	oat bran	barley porridge	Froot Loops
	porridge	Bran Buds	
		Bran Chex	
		cream of wheat	
		Healthwise	
		Just Right	
		Nutrigrain	
		instant porridge	
		Special K	

Medium GI (56–69)

FOODS	HEALTHY CHOICES	ENJOY OCCASIONALLY	UNHEALTHIER CHOICES
BREAKFAST CEREALS		Sustain	
CEREALS	basmati rice	boiled white rice	
	brown rice	corn taco shells	
	buckwheat	long-grain	
	corn meal	white rice	
	couscous	semolina	
PRESERVES AND SPREADS		apricot fruit spread	
		strawberry jam	
		honey	
CONFECTIONERY AND SNACKS		muesli bar	
			corn chips
			Mars bar
			potato crisps
			Snickers
			sports bars

Medium GI (56–69)

FOODS	HEALTHY CHOICES	ENJOY OCCASIONALLY	UNHEALTHIER CHOICES
LEGUMES		re-fried beans	
VEGETABLES	beetroot	boiled potatoes	
		canned potatoes	
		new potatoes	
		steamed potatoes	
		sweetcorn	
		sweet potatoes	
FRUIT	apricots, fresh	apricots, canned	
	cantaloupe melon	in syrup	
	kiwi fruit	fruit cocktail,	
	paw paw	canned	
	pineapple	peaches, canned	
	raisins	in syrup	
	sultanas		
FRUIT JUICE		cranberry juice	
		drink	

Medium GI (56–69)

FOODS	HEALTHY CHOICES	ENJOY OCCASIONALLY	UNHEALTHIER CHOICES
DAIRY DESSERTS			regular ice cream
MILK AND NON-DAIRY ALTERNATIVES			condensed milk
DRINKS		orange cordial	Cola Fanta orange other fizzy drinks*
CONVENIENCE FOODS	black bean soup green pea soup split pea soup	spaghetti bolognese	

High GI (70 and over)

FOODS	HEALTHY CHOICES	ENJOY OCCASIONALLY	UNHEALTHIER CHOICES
CAKES			doughnut
BISCUITS			Golden Fruit
			wafers
			corn thins
			puffed crispbread
			water biscuits
BREAD		buckwheat	bagel
		pancakes	baguette
		(gluten-free)	bread stuffing
			enriched white bread
			English muffin
			gluten-free bread
			kaiser rolls
			melba toast
			Middle-eastern flatbread

High GI (70 and over)

FOODS	HEALTHY CHOICES	ENJOY OCCASIONALLY	UNHEALTHIER CHOICES
BREAD			pikelets
			plain scones
			waffles
			white bread
PASTA AND NOODLES		corn pasta	
		rice pasta	
BREAKFAST CEREALS		Bran Flakes	Coco Pops
		Cheerios	corn flakes
		Grapenuts	Crunchy Nut
		Shredded Wheat	Corn Flakes
		Sultana Bran	Crispix
		wheat biscuits	Golden Grahams
		most cereal bars	Golden Wheats
			Honey Rice Bubbles
			Honey Smacks
			Pop Tarts

High GI (70 and over)

FOODS	HEALTHY CHOICES	ENJOY OCCASIONALLY	UNHEALTHIER CHOICES
BREAKFAST			Puffed Wheat
CEREALS			Rice Crispies
			Rice Chex
CEREALS		amaranth	
		glutinous (sticky)	
		rice	
		jasmine rice	
		millet	
CONFECTIONERY			fruit bars
AND SNACKS			jelly beans
			mint sweets
			popcorn
			Pop Tarts
			pretzels
			Skittles
			rice and corn
			snacks

High GI (70 and over)

FOODS	HEALTHY CHOICES	ENJOY OCCASIONALLY	UNHEALTHIER CHOICES
LEGUMES		broad beans	
VEGETABLES		baked potatoes	chips
		broad beans	instant mashed
		mashed potato	potato
		parsnips	
		pumpkin	
		swede	
FRUIT		dates	
		lychees	
		watermelon	
DAIRY DESSERTS		tofu-based frozen dessert	
DRINKS		*sports drinks:* Lucozade, Gatorade	

High GI (70 and over)

FOODS	HEALTHY CHOICES	ENJOY OCCASIONALLY	UNHEALTHIER CHOICES
DRINKS		Isostar; Sports Plus	
CONVENIENCE FOODS		pizza, tomato and cheese	

The step-by-step guide to easy low GI eating!

♥ Choose lower GI versions of the foods you usually eat, so eating healthily doesn't mean a complete overhaul of your diet. This will make it easier to stick to your decision to eat more healthily.

♥ Opt for wholegrain versions of foods, such as bread, rice and breakfast cereals.

♥ Look for foods that have undergone less processing, cooking or refining: choose boiled new potatoes in their skins instead of mashed potato, eat whole fruit instead of drinking juice and avoid over-cooking foods, especially vegetables. Even choose less ripe fruit, especially bananas.

♥ Swap high GI vegetables such as parsnips and pumpkin for lower GI veggies like leafy greens, peppers, aubergine and tomatoes.

♥ Combine high GI foods such as baked potatoes with a low GI food like baked beans to lower the overall GI of a meal.

♥ Read nutrition labels on foods and compare different types of foods to find those with higher fibre and lower sugar content.

♥ For best nutrition, keep those low GI but high fats foods to occasional, not everyday, treats.

♥ Limit your intake of sugary foods such as fizzy drinks and confectionery.

♥ If you do eat sugary treats, have these along with a main meal, so their glycaemic impact is lessened.

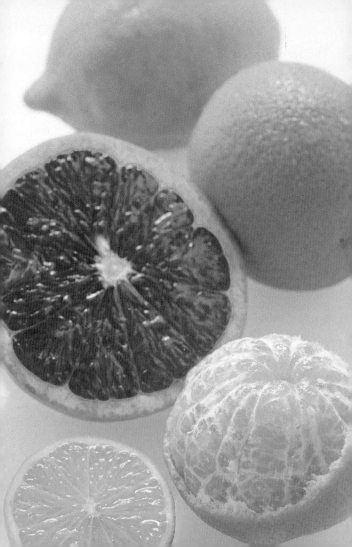

tools for a healthy body

Most of us will be able to tell when we've gained – or lost – a few pounds; the scales will let us know. How comfortable we feel in our clothes is another good indicator and, of course, the mirror never lies! If we gain weight, we might also feel sluggish or, somehow, just not quite ourselves. But it's easy to lose touch with what your weight means in terms of your health and where you are in relation to the healthy range. Yes, you might know that you weigh a little more than last year but what impact might that have on your health?

Knowing where your weight and other body measurements place you in terms of healthy ranges is a good place to start if you're wondering if you need to lose or gain weight, or can give you a bit of reassurance that your weight and body shape aren't negatively impacting on your health.

The tools in this chapter will help you find your body mass index (BMI), will let you know what your waist size means to your health and gives you information on the waist to hip ratio.

Another useful tool that, unfortunately, cannot be included here is body composition. Measuring percentage body fat can most easily be carried out using a technique called bioelectrical impedance. An electrical current is run through the body and since the current moves at different rates through muscle, fat and bone, the scale can calculate the proportions of fat to lean tissue. Many bathroom scales now come with this tool, and many larger scales found in chemists and even supermarkets also measure body fat.

Body composition can also be measured using hydrostatic weighing tanks or using calipers to measure skin-fold thickness, although these methods are only really used by professionals.

Healthy body fat ranges* are:		
	WOMEN (% fat)	MEN (% fat)
Essential fat	10–12%	2–4%
Athletes	14–20%	6–13%
Fitness	21–24%	14–17%
Acceptable	25–31%	18–25%
Obese	32% +	25% +

*According to the American Council on Exercise

Body Mass Index

BMI, or Body Mass Index, is a way to gauge our weight for height status. It can give us an idea if we are at a healthy weight, or below or above the healthy weight range for our height.

The normal healthy BMI range is categorized as being 20–25 (some agencies use 18.5–25); 26–30 is described as overweight; 30–40 is described as obese, while a BMI over 40 means that an individual is morbidly obese.

BMI can take only height and weight into consideration – it does not account for frame size or body composition. This means that BMI is not necessarily accurate for those of a very small or very large frame size, or those of a muscular or athletic build. It is also unsuitable for those under 18, over 65 or pregnant women.

Calculate your body mass index using the chart opposite. Locate your height in the right-hand (metres) or left-hand (feet) column of the chart then proceed across the top (for kilos) or the bottom (for stones). The number where these variables meet is your BMI.

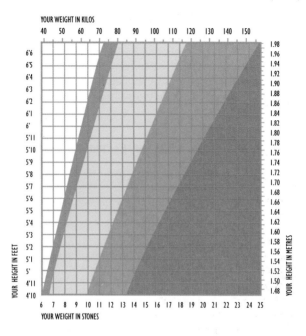

YOUR WEIGHT IN KILOS

YOUR HEIGHT IN FEET

YOUR HEIGHT IN METRES

YOUR WEIGHT IN STONES

CHART KEY

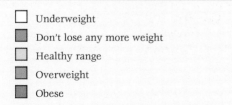

- [ ] Underweight
- [ ] Don't lose any more weight
- [ ] Healthy range
- [ ] Overweight
- [ ] Obese

Waist circumference

In cases when BMI is not appropriate, such as with athletes, another useful way to gauge weight and health status is using waist circumference. An increased waist measurement indicates abdominal obesity, that is, weight that accumulates around the trunk of the body. This 'apple' shape is associated with increased risk of diabetes and heart disease.

Risk of associated disease according to BMI and waist size			
BMI	Weight category based on BMI	Waist less than or equal to 40 in. (men) or 35 in. (women)	Waist greater than 40 in. (men) or 35 in. (women)
18.5 (20) or less	underweight	–	n/a
18.5 (20)–24.9	normal	–	n/a
25.0–29.9	overweight	increased	high
30.0–34.9	obese	high	very high
35.0–39.9	obese	very high	very high
40 or greater	morbidly obese	extremely high	extremely high

Waist to hip ratio

Another way to tell if you have an apple-shaped or pear-shaped body is the waist to hip ratio. To calculate your waist to hip ratio:

1   measure your waist around the navel
2   measure your hips around the buttocks
3   divide the waist measurement by the hip measurement

What do your results mean? Ratios above 0.8 in women and 0.95 in men mean that you have an apple shape.

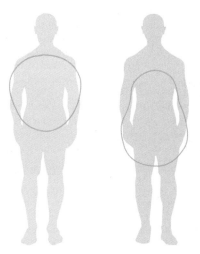

▲ *Those who carry weight around their trunk have an apple shape: this is associated with a greater risk of diabetes and heart disease than those with a pear shape, who carry extra weight around their hips.*

Q: Are there any negative side effects of following a low GI diet?

A: The only potential down-side of a low GI diet is that some low GI foods can be high in fat, since fat, fibre and protein all slow the rate at which carbohydrate foods are digested and so lower their GI value. But as long as we keep an eye on our fat intake and choose lower fat, low GI foods as the basis for our diet, this is perfectly healthy. There are no other known side effects or negatives to following the principles of GI.

Q: Will following the GI diet control my food cravings?

A: Yes! Cravings are often caused by a dip in blood sugar levels and when we eat low GI, we help to stabilize both blood sugars and our appetite. High GI foods, such as our morning bowl of corn flakes, are broken down quickly in the body and the sugars in these foods move quickly to the blood stream. This rise prompts the release of insulin, a hormone which acts to store that excess blood sugar away in fat cells, causing a fall in blood sugars. It's this fall that causes food cravings as the body tries to find a balance and level out blood sugar levels.

When we eat low GI foods, on the other hand, these are broken down much more gradually and don't promote the sugar highs and lows that cause food cravings. Low GI foods are also usually higher in fibre than high GI versions so these stay in the digestive system for longer and help us feel fuller for longer.

Another consequence of eating low GI is that we minimize insulin production – and insulin itself can act as an appetite stimulant.

Q: Can I follow the GI diet in conjunction with another diet?

A: As mentioned above, some low GI foods can be high in fat, such as nuts and chocolate. So when eating low GI, it's a good idea to think about your fat intake, too. The great thing about GI is that since you'll be eating wholegrain carbs, lean proteins, healthy fats and plenty of fruit and veg, you won't need to worry too much about fat – the foods you'll be choosing are the healthier options and soon you won't want to eat unhealthier, high fat foods like crisps or chips.

Apart from being aware of your fat intake, you won't need to follow GI principles in conjunction with any other diet – no grapefruits before every meal, no excluding of whole food groups and no need to eat weird and wonderful combinations of foods! You can throw those diet books away!

Q: What are the major sources of carbohydrates?

A: The main sources of carbohydrates in our diet are the foods we think of as 'fillers' – potatoes, bread, rice, pasta and cereals. Other important sources of complex carbs are legumes (peas, beans and lentils) and vegetables, especially root vegetables. The carbohydrates in fruit are mostly simple sugars, as are the carbs found in dairy products and, of course, sugary foods such as sweets, honey and preserves and baked goods like biscuits and cakes.

Complex carbs are our healthiest source of energy since these foods also provide a range of nutrients, for example, you'll find vitamin C and fibre in potatoes and B vitamins and minerals in bread. Sugary foods, on the other hand, provide only energy and are nutritionally void.

Q: I have a food intolerance – can I still follow the GI diet?

A: Yes, although you will need to modify the diet so suit your own personal needs. If you have an intolerance to wheat, for example, you'll need to replace pasta, bread and wheat-based breakfast cereals with other complex carbohydrates such as oats, brown rice, maize (corn) and new potatoes.

If you have a lactose intolerance and can't take dairy products, you can replace dairy foods with alternatives such as soy, rice or almond milk, tofu and other specialist non-dairy options. Do look for products that are fortified with calcium and vitamin D as dairy foods are our main source of these nutrients and choose other calcium-rich foods such as leafy green vegetables and beans.

So it is still possible to adapt the GI diet to your own requirements and the GI lists in this book will certainly help you find alternatives to particular foods you can't eat.

glossary

Amino acid the building blocks of proteins. There are 22 amino acids of which eight are essential, that is, must be supplied in the diet as they cannot be made in the body. These are tryptophan, lysine, methionine, phenylalanine, threonine, valine, leucine, isoleucine. Two others, histidine and arginine are essential only in children.

Anti-oxidant antioxidants are chemicals that prevent oxidation. Oxidation causes damage in the body, and is involved in ageing and the development of disease. Antioxidants combat this damage and help protect the body against disease. Antioxidant nutrients include vitamins A, C and E, selenium and beta-carotene.

Body mass index (BMI) used to give an indication of weight status in relation to height. BMI values of less than 18.5 are considered underweight, 19–25 is the healthy range, 26–29 is overweight, 30–39 is considered obese and 40+ is morbidly obese (see pages 146–47 for further information).

Calorie (kilocalorie) a unit of energy. The energy we derive from food is measured as kilocalories (usually abbreviated to 'calories') and kilojoules (kJ). One calorie equals 4.2 kJ. Fat provides 9 calories per gram, protein and carbohydrate each provide 4 calories per gram and alcohol provides 7 calories per gram (see page 11 for further information).

Carbohydrate a macronutrient that is used by the body as an energy source.

Cardiovascular disease diseases of the heart and blood vessels. Risk factors for cardiovascular disease include diabetes, metabolic syndrome, high blood pressure, high cholesterol and high triglyc-erides. These factors can all be modified through diet. Other modifiable risk factors are smoking and lack of exercise. Non-modifiable risk factors are age and genetic predisposition.

Cholesterol is a lipid sterol. It has functions in maintaining the stability of cell walls, in the synthesis of vitamin D and some hormones and immune function. Small amounts of cholesterol are found in the diet but most is made in the liver. Excess cholesterol is associated with cardiovascular disease.

Diabetes condition in which insulin function is impaired, either through an autoimmune disease that destroys insulin-producing cells (type 1 diabetes) or de-sensitization to insulin (type 2 diabetes) (see pages 31–32 for further information).

Diet the food we usually eat. Weight loss diets tend to change our eating habits; 'diet' is our habitual eating pattern.

Fat a macronutrient that is used as an energy source as well as being a carrier for fat-soluble vitamins (A, D, E and K) and a source of essential fatty acids.

Fatty acids components of fat (along with glycerol). Essential in the body for many functions, including brain development, nerve function, hormone regu-lation and even mood regula-tion.

Fibre polysaccharides that are complex in structure and cannot be digested by the body. Insoluble fibre protects the health of the digestive tract; soluble fibre helps lower choles-terol.

Free radical substances that cause oxidation. In the body, these active oxygen species can attack cells and DNA. Antioxidant nutrients mop up free radicals, limiting the damage they can cause.

Fructose a disaccharide with a GI value of around 19.

Glucose a monosaccharide. The body's preferred energy source, other saccharides are eventually metabolized to glucose for use in the body. Glucose is used as a reference to measure GI values of other foodstuffs.

Glycaemic index (GI) a scale showing the effects that different foods have on blood glucose levels, in relation to glucose itself.

Glycaemic load (GL) a measure of the impact carbo-hydrate foods have on the body, using both the glycaemic index and the amount of carbohy-drate found in foods (see page 65 for further information).

HDL cholesterol high density lipoprotein cholesterol – the healthy type of cholesterol that can help lower the risk of heart disease.

Hydrogenation a process that solidifies liquid vegetable oils. This increases shelf life of baked goods and can improve texture but it also creates trans fats, modified fats that have damaging effects on the body.

Insulin a hormone made in the pancreas that is used to regulate glucose levels.

LDL cholesterol low density lipoprotein cholesterol – the unhealthy type of cholesterol that increases the risk of heart disease.

Macronutrients essential nutri-ents that are needed in relatively large amounts: carbohydrate, protein and fat.

Metabolic syndrome a group of conditions that increases an individual's risk of diabetes and heart disease.

Micronutrients essential nutrients that are needed in relatively small amounts, including vitamins, minerals and phytonutrients.

Polyols sugar alcohols that add sweetness to food. These provide fewer calories than other carbohydrates and have low GI values.

Protein a macronutrient required for the growth and repair of the body.

Refining the process of removing the outer husk from grain to provide white grains such as white flour and rice. Removing the husk depletes the nutrient status of food and lowers the fibre content. Refined foods generally have higher GI values than their wholegrain equivalents.

Saccharide the building blocks of carbohydrates.

Wholegrain carbohydrate foods that include their husk. These provide more nutrients than refined versions, especially vitamins E and B, amino acids, magnesium, phosphorus and selenium.

REFERENCES

1. Jenkins DJ, Wolever TM, Taylor RH, Barker H, Fielden H, Baldwin JM, Bowling AC, Newman HC, Jenkins AL, Goff DV. *Glycaemic index of foods: a physiological basis for carbohydrate exchange*. Am J Clin Nutr. 1981;34(3):362–6.

2. Ebbeling CB, Ludwig DS. *Treating obesity in youth: should dietary glycaemic load be a consideration?* Adv Pediatr 2001;48:179–212.

3. Walton P, Rhodes EC. *Glycaemic index and optimal performance*. Sports Med 1997;23:164–72.

4. Frost G, Dornhorst A. *The relevance of the glycaemic index to our understanding of dietary carbohydrates*. Diabet Med 2000;17:336–45.

5. Willett W, Manson J, Liu S. *Glycaemic index, glycaemic load, and risk of type 2 diabetes*. Am J Clin Nutr 2002;76(suppl): 274S–80S.

6. Leeds AR. *Glycaemic index and heart disease*. Am J Clin Nutr 2002;76(suppl):286S–9S.

7. Brand-Miller JC, Holt SHA, Pawlak DB, McMillan J. *Glycaemic index and obesity*. Am J Clin Nutr 2002;76 (suppl):281S–5S.